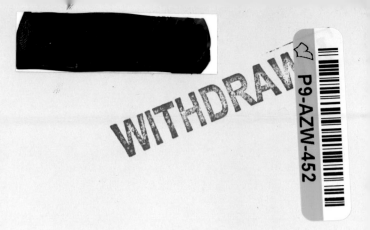
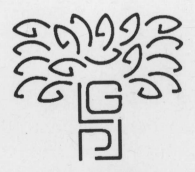

The
Lean

The
Lean

A Revolutionary (and Simple!) 30-Day
Plan for Healthy, Lasting Weight Loss

Kathy Freston

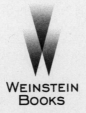

WEINSTEIN
BOOKS

ISBN: 978-1-60286-173-2 (hardcover)
ISBN: 978-1-60286-174-9 (e-book)

First Edition
10 9 8 7 6 5 4 3 2 1

The views expressed in this book are not intended as a substitute for professional medical advice.

I encourage you to seek the advice of your health-care provider before changing how you eat, especially if you have a serious medical condition. Check with your doctor to make sure you are advised to exercise; and as well, he or she may need to change (or even discontinue) medications because of the very powerful (and positive) effects of the modifications you are about to undertake in your diet. If you need to find a doctor, you might try contacting the American Holistic Medical Association for a referral, at 216-292-6644. You can also search their database at *http://www.holisticmedicine.org*.

Contents

Introduction

THERE'S SOMETHING ABOUT THE WORD *LEAN* THAT I ADORE, AND EVERY-where I go, other people seem to love it, too. In fact they kind of open up to it like flowers in sunshine—I think because it's such a mel-low word, an easy word. Nothing about it feels forced. My guess is you like the word too.

In my previous books, *Quantum Wellness* and *Veganist*, I talked about leaning in the direction of change and finding yourself mak-ing quantum changes in your lifestyle without much effort. In my own experience and the experience of the thousands of people who e-mail and tweet me about my books, talks, and TV appearances, weight loss is one of those changes that we can lean in to as well.

It's such a powerful concept, leaning.

Of course here we're playing with the word too. The double meaning is entirely intentional. This book is about getting lean in the bod, but it's also about leaning into weight loss so that it's not too difficult or overwhelming.

If you've read my other books, you know I'm all about ease. I like to do things with the least amount of effort to get the biggest pos-sible payoff. Don't you? If you've ever dieted, or if perhaps you've spent much of your life dieting, you've undoubtedly worked very,

very hard to achieve results. And possibly experienced the devastating shame or disappointment of having the weight creep back on. Whether you've been working against 10 pounds or 200, losing weight and keeping it off can be one of the toughest challenges, and I bow to you for the efforts you've made so far. What I'm here to tell you in this book, however, is that *it doesn't have to be hard.*

You read that right. Weight loss doesn't have to be hard. It's about setting an intention for what you want, weight- *and* healthwise, and then nudging yourself ever so gently in that direction. It's about making choices to eat foods that are delicious *and* filling *and* supportive of your weight loss goals. There is nothing in these pages that is drastic or strict, nothing that will require you to give up your favorite things altogether. Almost everything you'll find here has to do with taking steps away from the choices that made you heavy and toward choices that make you feel better. You will not feel denied and you will not be hard-pressed to get through the process. All I ask of you is your willingness to reach a little, your willingness to take just one step. And then another. To make small changes over time.

These little tweaks, like substituting soy or rice milk for cow's milk, for instance, or a handful of nuts for that bag of chips, will propel you almost effortlessly toward ever more healthy choices. You don't have to sacrifice favorite foods or family rituals. I'm talking about developing a different kind of friendship with food, not making it your enemy.

What you'll discover is that over time, not only do the little things add up, but they also work together synergistically to bolster your progress. We make so much possible just by adjusting and fine-tuning our meals and habits; so much is within our power to make better . . . one simple thing at a time.

Weight loss is not complicated. It doesn't require you to be a mathematician, calculating grams of protein and carbohydrates; you need not even understand what exactly body mass index is. It never made sense to me to focus on all those calculations, when it's so much simpler just to stay attuned to how we feel and look as a result of eating certain foods. Weight loss also doesn't require that you put yourself through physical drudgery and live in a constant state of longing or deprivation. That would not make a pleasant life, and no wonder so many of us reject, or fall down on, that hard-core path.

What you'll learn in the pages of this book is how to get into a natural rhythm of feeding your body what it thrives on, foods that are delicious, nutritious, and that inherently hold the secret of perfect balance and health. You'll also learn some new ways of thinking and relating that support the process. If you've had a kind of crazy love affair with certain foods, you may be called upon to face your obsessions, or even addictions—to sugar, cheese, etc. But you'll do this step by step, in stages, gently.

Here's the secret to this book: it's all about crowding out, not cutting out. *Crowding out* is a term used in nutritional circles to describe how to eat in a healthy way so that you never even have the chance to feel hungry. You literally crowd out the junk you think you want to eat by choosing to eat key foods throughout the day so that you're *always* satisfied. Isn't that preferable to depriving yourself of foods and white-knuckling it all the way?

> **Here's the secret to this book: it's all about crowding out, not cutting out.**

When you gradually add in nutrient-dense, fiber-rich foods, you simply stop feeling cravings. You run out of space in your belly for the old junk. Instead of craving, you feel full, fulfilled, content.

I'll tell you straight out: we are going to move away from eating animals and work in some delicious plant-based food, because as you'll see, the overwhelming amount of science and data say that this is the way to go if you want to lose weight healthfully *and* keep it off for good. You'll also be moving away from sugar and refined flours, but you'll have so much delicious and fulfilling food in the meantime, my strong hunch is that by the end of this program you won't even miss the old stuff. I'll go even farther and say that you're going to be floored to see the positive benefits to your weight loss and health when you really embrace this process.

Reader after reader has written to tell me how they simply dropped their extra weight by eating wholesome foods and getting the nasty (albeit sometimes delicious) stuff off their plates.

In the Lean, old bad habits get crowded out by better ones. It's the old switcheroo. But the key to the success of crowding out is doing it with a fair amount of ease. Diets that are too radically different from what we're used to generally don't work. That's because we want familiarity, tradition, hearty food, good taste. We don't want a whole new life; we want our same life, only absent a few (or more) pounds. If you listen closely, you might hear your true voice admitting, "I just don't want to give up the foods I love. Period." Fair enough, and who *does*? Not *moi*. Give up pizza for steamed broccoli and broiled chicken? No thanks. How about switching out pizza for pizza, though? Now we're talking, right? Jamessina, a reader who wrote to me, said, *"My childhood favorite meal was Mom's homemade beef stew. Now my husband cooks us his meatless chili, and it's incredible. It completely satisfies my craving for the texture and heartiness of the stew."*

What I'm here to tell you is that you can still eat your burgers and apple cobbler. Feeling excited yet? You should be! I'm going to introduce you to healthier versions of the things you grew up loving. Better yet, you'll have even more foods to choose from. Yep, that's right—more food!

Here's how it works: I'm going to have you *add* healthier choices to whatever else you're already eating. All I ask is that you eat (or do) the new stuff first. That's the only catch. Before you dig into whatever it is you really want to eat, you're going to have a few whole grains and beans and fruits and veggies and nuts (et cetera, et cetera, et cetera!). And then I'm going to tell you how to make some simple switches.

It's a double whammy that will do quite a number on your waistline. Gradually. Easily. No white knuckles.

Aside from substantial and lasting weight loss (as if that weren't enough), here's what you can expect from doing this:

- more energy
- a general feeling of increased wellness
- more menu options
- brighter skin
- improved digestion

Satiety. Satisfaction. Fullness.

As you lean in to this healthier way of eating, not only will your taste buds change, but you will too. You will stop wasting time caught up in a tug of war between cravings and guilt. You will be freed up to work toward your life's purpose, whatever that purpose may be. (I can assure you, your life's purpose is not to fret about eating the doughnuts, eating them, shaming yourself for eating them, and then acting out by eating more. Or undertaking a grueling diet for payback.)

The more you lean in to healthy eating, the more you will be supported by feelings of well-being—not just in your body, but in your mind and soul, too.

Within us all is the impulse to grow and evolve, to transcend who we are today and become a clearer, brighter version of ourselves. To do that, we have to shed the weight, literally and metaphorically. This shift doesn't happen overnight, and it shouldn't. It took a lifetime to get where you are, and if you try to lose pounds super quickly, they probably won't stay off. You'll get bored, or you'll crave the old yummies, or you'll go out of your mind with rules, rules, rules. But when you make changes little by little—changes to what you eat and how you think—your body will kick into gear and the weight will begin to come off without much effort. You will soar.

How many pounds, and how fast? Truthfully, weight and health are so much more about how you feel and look than about a number on a scale. But here's the skinny: Once the process is in full gear, at the end of the 30 days, you can expect to lose between 1 and 3 pounds a week. Compared with a fad diet that may not sound like a lot, but it really is quite substantial, and even better, safe. Although you might certainly lose more than this, this rate of loss allows your body to get comfortable with new regimens and eases you into your new lifestyle. And that's what *sustainable* weight loss is all about. Slow, steady, uncomplicated, and lasting. No matter what your weight loss goal—whether it's 200 pounds (like Natala, whom you will hear from later) or 100 pounds (like her husband, Matt), the Lean can help you get there—all you need to do is keep on leaning, and before you know it, you will be transformed.

We'll get your body moving and feeling strong, too; but we'll do it as you're ready, and in a way that is approachable and comfortable. And because I believe that the body and mind are intricately connected, I'm going to give you some tweaks to *think* about—ways to subtly shift your emotional stance. These little mental adjustments might just prove to be the magic that brings the whole plan together, and you need do nothing but keep your mind open and your heart willing.

Simply lean in to change where it's possible and before you know it, you will be on the path to slim.

The Lean: How It Works

Here's how the Lean plan works. Every day for 30 days, I'm going to give you one new thing to do, something to tweak in your daily routine. Some days you'll be adding new foods and others you'll be switching out one food for another. There will also be assignments that have to do with fulfilling emotional needs, because again, it's not just about food itself.

Along the way you'll hear about people's experiences with weight loss—truly inspiring stories. Some of the people you'll meet leaned in gradually, while some of them ran with the changes they learned about. Some were inspired by books they read or a film they watched, while others had health issues that spurred them to make changes. All of them found their way in the manner that was right for them, at the speed that made sense for their particular situation. These snippets of stories are meant to show you that no matter where you are on the spectrum of weight and health, there is a way through that will deliver you to success.

Each day builds on the previous one, so what you do on Day 1 you will *also* do on Day 2 and Day 3 and so on, along with the new tweaks. By the end of the 30 days you will have 30 new habits. Small, manageable, easy changes. Changes that move you toward plant-based foods, which are indisputably the best for you, and away from sugar and fat. You won't mind the changes at all, not only because they're small, easy, and delicious, but because the weight will start melting off. And it all starts with taking just one step and leaning in the direction of change.

> **Each day builds on the previous one, so what you do on Day 1 you will *also* do on Day 2 and Day 3 and so on, along with the new tweaks.**

What you'll want to do is *read each day's Lean the day before you actually do it* so that you're prepared with groceries or whatever else you might need. Read through it again as you are making the change to make sure you've digested it. With each successful day, check off the tweak from the list that you'll see at the end of each chapter to ensure you haven't forgotten anything. If you miss a day for some reason, just pick up where you left off the next day, do everything asked of you on the checklist, and then move on.

A true lifestyle change means slowly adapting to healthier behaviors in everyday living, so if this day plan is going a bit too fast, feel free to stretch it out to a more comfortable schedule. You could, for instance, do one tweak per week or month rather than one per day, or you could simply move to the next step in the plan as you feel ready. The schedule and speed are entirely up to you; what's important is that you are leaning in to being healthier and more fit!

You are about to be transformed, one slight shift at a time. Enjoy this wonderful ride!

The
Lean

DAY 1.

Drink Water. Lots of Water.

Remember to read this a day ahead so you're ready to begin!

THIS IS IT. THE BIG DAY. DAY 1 OF YOUR WEIGHT LOSS LEAN, ONE EASY, gradual, pleasurable step at a time. Well, breathe a big sigh of relief, because today is going to be super easy. You can relax and keep eating everything you are used to. (Do I hear cheering? Audible exhales?) No need to cut anything out or limit your intake or weigh your food. You don't even have to bring anything special to work or push yourself to move your bod.

Nope, the only thing I want you to do today is drink water.

Sounds too easy, eh? Well, sometimes the greatest gifts are right underneath our nose, and in this case, it's in the glass you raise to your lips.

Water is so purifying, so cleansing. You might even think of this tweak as a way to wash away your past problems with weight so that you can start afresh. A purification or cleansing of your body.

There's more to it than that, of course, and don't think for a second that I'm going to ask you to make changes without giving you the science to support them. Fear not. We'll get there. But today is about just one thing: drinking water.

I want you to be methodical about this to be absolutely sure you are getting the full benefit, so here's how we're going to do this.

First thing when you wake up, drink an 8-ounce glass of room temperature water. Have the glass waiting by your bedside so that you can just roll over, pick it up, and swig it down. (Okay, maybe you should sit up first so you don't spill it all over yourself!)

Get out of bed, do what you need to—shower, get dressed, wake the kids, gear up for breakfast. About 10–20 minutes before breakfast, swig down another big glass of water. Juice does not count. Coffee does not count. (Now, don't freak out. This doesn't mean you can't drink coffee too; you can. It just means that water means water.)

I say swig—or gulp—it down because this way you actually get the volume I'm looking for. If you are sipping, you may not get around to drinking the entire glass. And if you are not usually a water drinker, every sip might just be arduous. That said, there are some who say that if you don't sip slowly, the water just drains right out of you, like when you overwater a plant rather than giving it just enough—and slowly enough so that it's absorbed. But for now, to get you into the habit, simply knock back the glasses. You can sip throughout the day on top of what I tell you to drink, but let's just be sure to get your eight 8s out of the way.

Extra Lean: Add some freshly squeezed lemon juice to your water first thing in the morning for the added benefit of antioxidants and phytonutrients—phytonutrients like limonin that have slowed the growth of colon cancer and HIV in petri dish experiments. Plus, a squeeze of lemon makes it taste good!

Then, somewhere between breakfast and lunch, say around 9:30 or 10 A.M., have another glass. And another ten or twenty minutes before lunch. Number five between lunch and dinner. Another right before dinner. Number seven a couple of hours after dinner. And the final glass right before you go to bed. You can have more if you are thirsty after a workout or on a hot day, or whenever you feel the need.

How could you possibly be thirsty with all that water, you might ask. Funny thing, but drinking begets thirst, and even if this is way more water than you are used to, you will find yourself thirsting for more. I know that when I get out of the habit, I have to really push myself to drink. I don't think I'm thirsty, and I don't particularly like the taste (as if water had a taste). But once in the swing, I want even more. Trust me, it's just a matter of creating the habit.

Extra Lean: Most water actually does have a taste, albeit a subtle one, and depending on your source you may not like that taste very much. Water's taste is affected by its source and even by the pipes it runs through. If you don't like the taste of your tap water, you might want to get a filter—anything from a pitcher with a built-in filter to a simple system that attaches to your tap to a more elaborate one that has to be hooked up by a handyperson or plumber. You'll really notice the difference in flavor.

Personally, I'd stay away from bottled water unless you absolutely have to go that route to find water you'll drink. Bottled waters are expensive, and they're generally no healthier than tap (in fact, bottled water is less strictly regulated for chemical and microbial contamination, and on top of that, the plasticizing compounds found in many water bottles have been shown to have negative health effects). Not to mention that a lot of resources are wasted in the production of plastic and glass.

No doubt you've heard that water is good for you, and you should drink lots of it to stay hydrated so your cells function optimally. But did you know that drinking water can actually be a powerful aid to weight loss? A 2010 study published in the journal *Obesity* found that drinking 17 ounces of water (about 2 cups) before each main meal (a practice known as "pre-loading" in clinical circles) helped significantly reduce participants' caloric intake. Along with calorie reduction, participants who drank 2 cups of water before meals lost an average of 5 pounds of fat *more* than those who didn't over the course of the twelve-week study.

Water and Metabolism

These results may have occurred because the water simply filled up the stomach (a volumetric benefit) and subsequently reduced overall calorie intake (Because there is only so much room in the belly, after all!). But staying hydrated also keeps your body's biological processes working at their fullest potential, and this includes your metabolism—something you want to work as well as possible when you're trying to shed excess weight. Here's the science of metabolism: metabolism is both catabolism (harvesting energy by breaking down compounds like fats and protein) and anabolism (using that energy to build stuff, like our own fats and proteins). Or more simply, it's the breaking down of foods to use as energy and building material. It's the culmination of many biological processes, of which water is an absolutely essential component.

> Staying hydrated also keeps your body's biological processes working at their fullest potential, and this includes your metabolism.

Hydration is critical because it keeps your metabolism working efficiently and helps keep your metabolic rate up. You'll burn more calories during the day if you're hydrated. Dehydration, on the other hand, makes your metabolic rate slow down, and may even make you feel less energetic. A University of Utah researcher has claimed that those who drank water according to the 8 x 8 recommendation (eight 8-ounce glasses per day) reported increased concentration and energy and a higher resting metabolic rate. The rise in metabolic rate achieved by drinking water is modest, and works best in conjunction with other simple lifestyle changes (which we will get to in the coming days), but it is one small thing you can do to speed up or maintain weight loss. A few small changes in your daily routine can pay huge dividends to your health. Plus, drinking plenty of water minimizes the space in your diet for sodas, sweet fruit juices, or other empty liquid calories; you might very likely even lose the taste for unhealthy drinks.

And there are two more benefits to drinking water: decreased fluid retention and the more efficient removal of cellular waste from your body. See, I told you this would be purifying! Drinking lots of water discourages your body from holding on to water weight. This is even truer for a menstruating woman. The more you drink, the more you will pee, and the lighter you will begin to feel. Additionally, adequate water intake ensures that your kidneys can perform properly, and one of the essential functions of the kidneys is to remove from your body the wastes from the metabolic process via the urinary tract.

The Institute of Medicine, an independent, nonprofit organization, recommends 11 to 12 cups, or about 91 ounces, of water per day for women (men need about 13 cups). Their recommendation goes up for pregnant (12–13 cups) and breastfeeding women (16 cups!), by the way. Don't be intimidated by this number; while it may sound like quite a lot, with a healthy diet you'll obtain about 20 percent of this from the food you eat. The question, then, is how much water *should* you be drinking independent of your food intake? The 8 x 8 rule is easy to remember, and adds up to 64 ounces per day.

Fortunately, it's not expensive or difficult to achieve this goal. You can buy a reusable water bottle or canteen (steel is best, or BPA-free plastic) or a pitcher if you work at a desk, and aim for filling it up and emptying it 3 to 4 times per day (most hold 20–24 ounces).

And in general, the larger and more active you are, the more water you'll need. You can monitor how you are doing in terms of being well hydrated by looking at the color of your urine: if it's light to clear, you are well hydrated; if it's the color of apple juice or darker, you are probably dehydrated and need to drink more. (Note: supplements of certain vitamins, such as riboflavin, will artificially darken your urine.)

A little note here: don't get crazy on me with too much water. Too much of anything is not a good thing, water included. You can actually get overhydrated if you drink way in excess of the recommendation, thereby flushing out the electrolytes in your body; lack of electrolytes can produce fatal disturbance in brain function. Again, you'd have to drink way more than the eight 8s, so this is just a warning to those of you who might want to take things to the extreme. Don't be extreme; remember, we're all about leaning and natural ease!

So there you go, Day 1! Just drink your water—at least 8 ounces, 8 times a day, before you drink or eat your regular fare. And that's all!

DAY 2.

Have a Hearty Breakfast

WELCOME TO DAY 2!

Yesterday you hydrated really well, and today you'll be doing that too. And of course now we're adding something new: a nice big dish of love first thing in the morning. Yep, today is about starting the day with a hearty and healthy breakfast.

Okay, I know you've heard it before, but it's true. Breakfast *is* the most important meal of the day. When you feed yourself what your body needs when it needs it, that's love. So give your bod some TLC and sit down and enjoy a good, substantial breakfast.

To some this may sound counterintuitive. Doesn't skipping breakfast cut down on calories?

Short answer? No.

You actually need the calories first thing in the morning to jump-start your metabolism. Skipping them will do you no good, as you will only be hungrier and eat more later. Hunger and self-control do not go hand in hand.

Here's why: When you skip food for a long period of time, your body goes into starvation mode. Your blood sugar drops,

> **When you skip food for a long period of time, your body goes into starvation mode.**

7

you get cranky, and you can't think straight. Your body doesn't know what's going on or when it will get food, so it slows down the metabolism—by as much as 40 percent—in order to hold on to what it does have. You don't want that! What you want is to rev up your metabolism so that you are burning fat and calories, not preserving fat and calories. Not eating breakfast leads to overeating later on in the day. In fact, research shows that a common characteristic of obese people is that they tend to skip breakfast.

Skipping food slows down the metabolism— by as much as 40 percent.

And when I say eat breakfast, I'm not talking about some measly hard-boiled egg! No dry toast with grapefruit juice. No siree! I'm talking a bowl of steel-cut oatmeal or hot cream of rice cereal. Or a couple of pieces of whole grain toast smeared with peanut or almond butter. Or if you are the savory sort, go for some scrambled tofu with sweet potatoes and salsa. I've got some great suggestions in the recipe section.

You see, when you eat a good breakfast of complex carbs, like those in steel-cut oats or brown rice or whole grain bread, you get a slow and steady release of glucose that powers your body for hours. That's right. Eat a power breakfast and it will carry you through to lunch with no midmorning slump. And it'll put your body on course for weight loss by helping you burn calories all day.

It's so simple, really: it's all about the fiber.

The one dietary component most highly and consistently associated with long-term weight loss is fiber consumption.

In all the medical literature, the one dietary component most highly and consistently associated with long-term weight loss is fiber consumption. The customary reason offered for why fiber helps us control our weight is that it adds volume to foods, yet yields zero calories since, by definition, fiber is not something that we can digest. It's like we talked about on Day 1—if you drink a glass of water every time before you eat, you'll feel full quicker because some of your stomach volume is taken up by calorie-free water. Well, you can think of fiber as water in food form. Health benefits without any calories.

> ***Extra Lean:*** Did you know that foods filled with fiber—whole grains, beans, legumes, veggies—reduce your levels of C-reactive protein, which rise in response to inflammation in your body? It's good to get your inflammation down, as most degenerative diseases begin as inflammatory processes, and inflammation fattens your body.

Think about it this way. The average stomach can hold about a quart of food. If we filled that quart with bacon and eggs, it would yield more than 5,000 calories (5,329 to be exact), a few days' worth all in a single meal. The same amount of oatmeal would make you feel just as full (even more so, actually, since it would sponge up water in your stomach and expand further), but at a small fraction of the calories.

Obesity is so rare among those eating high-fiber diets that nutrition researchers have been desperate to uncover their secret. Yes, dietary records show high-fiber eaters do tend to eat fewer calories (you can't stuff as much in because your belly is full!), but not *that* many fewer. So what's going on?

Obesity is so rare among those eating high-fiber diets that nutrition researchers have been desperate to uncover their secret.

Scientists have put forth a number of theories. There is exciting new research, too, suggesting that the benefits of fiber extend beyond its bulk.

Here's what Michael Greger, M.D., founder of Nutrition Facts.org, a peer-reviewed science-based website, says:

A lot of it might have to do with the fact that people eating high-fiber diets have been found to burn more calories because they express more of the enzyme (carnitine palmitoyltransferase) that shovels fat into the furnaces (mitochondria) in our cells. Maybe it's because of the obesogens—endocrine-disrupting industrial chemical pollutants in the meat supply—they're avoiding. Maybe obesity-causing animal viruses in meat (like the chicken adenovirus SMAM-1) are even playing a role.

But maybe it's also the propionate, a compound produced from the digestion of fiber. After all, what's one of the things that's only in plant foods, never in animal foods? Fiber. Each cell wall surrounding each plant cell is made out of fiber. Animals don't have cell walls (we just have cell membranes) and so there is no fiber found in any products derived from animals. Animals have bones to hold them up; plants (like oats or rice or wheat or nuts) have fiber to hold them up. Just as plants don't contain bones, animals don't contain fiber.

How can propionate be a product of fiber digestion? Didn't I just say that fiber was defined by our inability to digest it? True, we can't digest it, but the gazillions of good bacteria in our guts can. What do they make with it? Propionate, which then gets absorbed into our bloodstream from our large intestine. So technically we can digest fiber, but just not without a little help from our little friends.

What does propionate do? It appears to have a "hypophagic effect," meaning it helps us eat less by apparently slowing down the rate at which food empties from our stomachs, thereby making us feel full longer. In addition to helping regulate food intake, propionate may also suppress the generation of new fat cells, resulting in an overall anti-obesity effect.

A note here about whole grains (like oats or brown rice) versus refined carbs (such as white bread and many boxed cereals): we call whole grains or complex carbohydrates "good carbs" because they are still in their natural state with all the fiber included. When you eat whole grains, the fiber causes your food to be digested and absorbed into your bloodstream slowly. This helps to keep your blood sugar in a normal range without getting too high or too low, thus no wild cravings. But when whole grain flour is processed, or "refined," into white flour, or ground to make cereal crisps, the beneficial fiber and bran are either altogether or somewhat removed. You want to eat "good carbs" rather than "bad carbs" so that you *feel steady, full, and satiated.*

Personally, I enjoy a bowl of brown rice for breakfast most of the time. I make a big pot of it (I actually use a rice cooker, which is super easy and involves practically no cleanup) twice a week and keep it in the fridge. I scoop out about 2 cooked cups worth of rice, chop up some apples or dried apricots and walnuts, sprinkle some cinnamon, and pour on some heated unsweetened almond, soy, or rice milk with a tad of agave nectar to sweeten it a bit. It's delicious and it keeps me satisfied and energized for hours as the unrefined carbohydrates slowly break down in my system.

Extra Lean: Sprinkle some cinnamon on your food; it reduces your blood sugar levels and increases insulin sensitivity so that you feel more steady and satiated.

Many Chinese people have rice for breakfast (it's called congee or *juk*, and it's like a gruel or porridge; it can be made sweet or savory). I mention the Chinese because they usually eat rice three times a day, and you don't see many overweight Chinese people, especially those in the countryside who have not been exposed to the Western way of eating. They eat lots of carbs (they even eat white rather than brown rice) and they are *still* slim. I, too, enjoy rice throughout the day. Sometimes I will use what I have stored in the fridge as a side dish for lunch or dinner (sautéed veggies and chickpeas go great on top, as does grilled veggie sausage or black beans and avocado, for instance). Later still, I might enjoy mixing in some hot vanilla or hazelnut soy creamer with raisins and cinnamon for a hearty and delicious dessert. Okay, enough about rice; I just wanted to share with you how versatile and useful it is!

Back to breakfast! Many people equate breakfast with eggs, and you've probably noticed that I haven't recommended them. Let's talk about eggs for a moment. The primary problem with eggs from a weight loss standpoint is that they have absolutely no fiber, and that's not good for your metabolism. But let's also take a look at what eating eggs does to your health: I know you are aware of how widespread heart disease and stroke is, and cholesterol is a big part of the problem. Well, did you know that one egg has as much cholesterol as an 8-ounce steak? One egg has more cholesterol than a double Quarter Pounder with cheese, and eating one or more per day ups your risk of type 2 diabetes by 77 percent for women and 58 percent for men (this from a 2008 study of more than 57,000 people).

Another study, the Nurses' Health Study, was conducted at Harvard University beginning in 1976 with funding from the National Institutes of Health, and enrolled more than 100,000 women. As you can imagine, with a sample size that large it is now considered the most definitive long-term study ever on older women's health. In that time thousands have died, but earlier this year the authors published their definitive risk factors for mortality analysis. The number one cause of death was heart disease, and cholesterol consumption was a significant risk factor for death. The second leading cause of death was smoking-related cancer. Comparing the two, a woman who consumes the amount of cholesterol found in a single egg a day cuts her life expectancy by as much as she would if she smoked five cigarettes a day for fifteen years.

And if that's not enough to sway you from eggs, a new National Institutes of Health–sponsored study appeared in September of 2011, reporting that men who eat 2.5 eggs or more per week have an 81 percent higher chance of developing lethal prostate cancer. Yikes. I'd opt for steel-cut oats or toast and peanut butter any old day!

On the other side of the coin, the most health-protective behavior researchers found was fiber consumption. Eating just a cup of oatmeal a day appears to extend a woman's life span as much as if she jogged four hours a week! (Of course there's no reason why you can't do both, and we'll get to that soon.) And here are a few things you may not know: cholesterol is found only in animal foods (there is essentially zero cholesterol in nonanimal food) and is significantly associated with living a shorter life, whereas fiber, which is found only in plant foods, is significantly associated with living longer. Okay, so you can see why I'm axing eggs in favor of oatmeal!

My half-sister, Kathy, leaned into her 30-pound weight loss, and now she and her kids eat dairy- and egg-free waffles sweetened with agave syrup (more about agave on Day 23) or a banana, and topped with slivered almonds. Not so tough a transition, eh? See how easy this can be?

Now, if you want to kick your metabolism up a notch, add some plant protein to your breakfast. Whole grains are a good source of protein themselves, but the Brits and Aussies may be on to something by eating beans for breakfast. Dr. Greger explains: "When food hits our small intestine, there are specific receptors on nerves in our gut that send satiety signals to our brain that make us feel full, and the presence of protein may help us feel more satiated. Protein is also harder for our bodies to process, which means that the body has to expend extra energy to break it down (the so-called "thermic effect")—good news if we're trying to burn every extra calorie we can." You could sprinkle a small handful of almonds or walnuts on your oatmeal, or have a scoop of protein powder shaken with water, or a side of veggie sausages to achieve this extra burn.

You might be noticing already, astute reader, that I'm a big fan of foods that are grown in the ground or on trees, and I want to nudge you more toward eating them. Plant-based foods like whole grains, sweet potatoes, beans and lentils, veggies, and fruits are chock-full of nutrition and fiber, while animal foods are chock-full-a trouble: saturated fat and zero fiber, and they cause all kinds of health problems. The fewer animals and animal products you eat, the better. But don't worry, we'll get into that soon enough!

So, what are you going to do today?

- ✓ Drink lots of water.
- ✓ Eat a hearty breakfast.

DAY 3.

Eat an Apple

TODAY, I WANT YOU TO ENJOY AN APPLE. CUT IT IN QUARTERS OR CHOP it up in bites, or just grab it and go.

(Water, a hearty breakfast, and now apples? So far, so good, right?)

Apples are so common you've probably forgotten how absolutely delicious they are, so pure and sweet and crunchy. There is something clean about an apple, so elementally uncomplicated and straightforward. I always buy a big bag of apples once a week at the farmers' market and keep them on my kitchen counter as a centerpiece. Nice to be able to munch on the centerpiece, don't you think? I keep them there as a reminder to dig in, and also as a counterweight should I get itchy for a sweet snack. If I'm rooting around for something to eat, I'll grab an apple while I'm looking, and usually by the time I'm finished eating it, my hunger has been sidelined. Crowding out at its best! Anyway, you can have it in the midmorning, in the afternoon, or before bed; it's entirely up to you. But before the day's end, you must eat an apple. Not apple juice or applesauce (and certainly not apple pie or an apple muffin!). Just a good ol' whole apple. Any kind will do.

Why is eating an apple part of the Lean plan?

15

We've all the heard the old adage "An apple a day keeps the doctor away." But there is new evidence that this single daily apple has significant, measurable benefits. A major review published in 2008 out of the German Cancer Research Center found that indeed, compared with those who eat less than an apple a day, those who eat one or more had less risk of oral cancer, cancer of the voice box, breast cancer, and colon, kidney, and ovarian cancer as well.

This makes sense given new research from Cornell University showing that apple peels had potent antioxidant and growth-blocking effects on human breast cancer cells examined in a petri dish, and the higher the apple concentration, the fewer the cancer cells. And apples seem to work best against estrogen-receptor-negative breast cancer, which is much harder to treat than the receptor-positive kind.

How do apples do what they do?

There are three stages of tumor formation. Carcinogens cause the initial DNA mutations (the initiation stage), and then oxidation, inflammation, and hormones cause it to grow (the promotion stage); finally, metastasis occurs, in which the cancer spreads throughout the body. Which steps have apples been found to block? *All* of them. Apples not only have antimutagenic, antioxidant, and anti-inflammatory effects, but they may even enhance our immune systems to help clear out any budding tumors before they get their start.

But in addition to boosting your immune system, that apple has other benefits that can help you lose weight. Surprised? Here we go, back to fiber.

Most Americans don't get enough fiber each day to meet their nutritional requirements. It's recommended that women get at least 25 grams of fiber per day on a 2,000-calorie diet, or to be more precise, 14 grams of fiber per 1,000 calories consumed. However, the average American only gets about 15 grams daily. Twenty-five grams is actually at the low end of your optimal fiber intake, so there's no reason not to aim higher. We humans actually evolved eating more than 100 grams of fiber a day, largely from wild greens. So back to that apple: How does an apple measure up in terms of fiber? Eating just one apple a day (skin on) will give you on average 4.4 grams of fiber.

Eating just one apple a day (skin on) will give you on average 4.4 grams of fiber.

You know by now that eating a high-fiber diet is beneficial for a whole host of physical reasons, including the prevention of many diseases and a clogged-up colon, but you're not alone if you're unsure what exactly to eat to reach that daily fiber goal. Fortunately, eating enough of the right foods is really rather simple, especially on the Lean plan, since I'll be introducing so many whole grains, beans and lentils, and veggies into your daily routine. And there will be even more space on your plate for high-fiber foods once you cut back on less-nutritious animal protein (which has no fiber at all, zero, zilch), but we'll get to that later.

If you're uncertain what 25 grams of fiber looks like, or if that sounds like a lot, consider the ease of incorporating the following into your daily diet:

- ¼ cup of cooked steel-cut oats (4 grams)
- ½ cup of cooked beans (10 grams)
- *1 apple with skin (3–5 grams)*
- ½ cup of vegetables (4 grams or more, depending on the vegetable; some are higher in fiber than others)

As you can see, a single apple is an easy and delicious way to get up to a fifth of your recommended 25 grams of fiber daily.

Again, don't rely on apple juice, or any fruit juices in general, to get fiber. You get all the sugar in the juice, but none of the fiber. Chewing is key. A 2011 study from the school of public health at Harbin Medical University in China shows chewing may help our bodies regulate the amount of food we take in, and in fact, may cause us to consume about 12 percent fewer calories per meal than if we wolf down our food without chewing carefully. Not only does chewing well slow down our consumption and give our body time to feel full, but it also assists the body in absorbing more nutrients. There are internal sensors in the gut that tell the brain when we have had enough food with enough nutrients, and when we are sated, the hunger message turns off. The scientists who conducted the study wrote in their paper that "mastication apparently plays a role in the gut hormone profile, which consequently influences energy [caloric] intake."

Another study relevant to our discussion on taking your time with chewing was published in 2011 in the *Journal of the American Dietetic Association*; in it, researchers found that people who ate fast were more likely to be overweight than people who ate slowly. Good thing that the high-fiber food featured in the Lean plan encourages us to take longer with every bite!

> **Researchers found that people who ate fast were more likely to be overweight than people who ate slowly.**

The feeling of hunger is very much influenced by hormonal signals, and the hormone ghrelin particularly. I think of ghrelin like the hunger gremlin; it pushes and grumbles for more food. Researchers found that when study participants chewed more, their ghrelin levels were reliably lower after meals. So, the longer food is chewed, the less ghrelin is released, and the longer you feel satiated. Now, *that's* something to chew on!

How many chews, you might ask? In the experiment, participants who chewed 40 times rather than 15 times consumed fewer calories; but I'd rather you not worry about counting your chews. The point is that when you eat high-fiber whole foods, you must chew. By their very nature, the foods require that you masticate well before swallowing.

And before we move on from hormones, a study at the University of California–Davis in 2002 found that eating fiber causes the release of a hormone in the stomach called cholecystokinin, and that hormone plays a direct role in letting your brain know that you are fine, that you got what you need.

In so many ways, fiber is critical for healthy weight loss. It makes us feel full and satiated, turns off the hunger signal, and it also cleans out our bodies like a powerful internal scrub brush. I have a friend who used to be constipated for a week at a time; she thought she ate well and avoided fatty foods, but she never quite got around to eating fruits. She started eating an apple a day (sometimes even two or three) and now her bowels move twice a day. (Once is just fine, by the way; let's call the second time a bonus!) Her tummy flattened out, her skin took on a glow, and she has a lot more energy without that stuffed-up, compacted feeling she used to walk around with.

Extra Lean: Have a doctor check your hormones to make sure everything is working properly; if your thyroid is off, it will be nearly impossible to lose weight. Other signs that your thyroid is out of whack are general lethargy, dry hair and skin, and brittle nails.

On top of that, apples are a rich source of a particularly powerful type of fiber called pectin. It's what's used as a gelling agent to make jams and jellies, and in our stomach it can delay stomach emptying through a similar mechanism. Researchers at UCLA showed that by swapping in pectin for regular fiber they could double the time it took subjects' stomachs to empty from about 1 hour to 2 hours, which meant subjects felt full that much longer. In fact there was even a study entitled "Weight Loss Associated with a Daily Intake of Three Apples or Three Pears among Overweight Women" published in the journal *Nutrition*. Researchers found that instructing women to eat an apple or pear before each meal resulted in significant weight loss.

Researchers found that instructing women to eat an apple or pear before each meal resulted in significant weight loss.

Pretty cool, no? They were told, in

effect, to eat more food, to add the fruit on top of their regular diets, and what happened was, the fruit crowded out less healthy choices; they ended up eating fewer calories overall and they started shedding pounds.

Other great sources of this superfiber include citrus, peaches, peas, and carrots. So yes, you can have an apple. Or a pear. Or an orange. You can even have two or three. But at the very least, have an apple before the day is done.

So what are you going to do today?

✓ Drink lots of water.
✓ Eat a hearty breakfast.
✓ Eat an apple!

DAY 4.

Clean Out the Cupboards, and Just for Today, Say No to Your Poison

YOU'VE BEEN AT THIS FOR THREE DAYS NOW, AND IT HASN'T BEEN HARD at all, right? More water, a hearty breakfast, an apple—easy stuff. But I know as well as anyone does that a lot of us have foods we simply can't resist, and we haven't really touched on those at all. Today is all about how to successfully avoid our particular poisons.

I need to tell you something: There's a reason you can't resist certain foods even though you know they're no good for you and even though you have an intense desire to lose weight. It's not about your lack of willpower or terrible moral weakness, it's about specific biological processes that set intense cravings into motion. In other words, it's biological. It's not your fault! So you can stop beating yourself up and start feeling a little better about yourself.

What researchers have found is that the craving for certain foods comes from primitive neurochemical reward (or feel-good) centers in the brain that dominate normal willpower and beat out our ordinary biological signals that control hunger. In simple terms, fat and sugar trigger your brain to push you to eat more! Your brain is looking for nutrients,

Your brain is looking for nutrients, not calories, so if you aren't getting the nutrients, your brain says keep going.

not calories, so if you aren't getting the nutrients, your brain says keep going.

Sugar and fat stimulate the brain's reward centers through the neurotransmitter dopamine, exactly like other addictive drugs do. When we eat fatty or sugary foods, we are flooded with that feel-good brain chemical. (Heroin and morphine work much the same way; dopamine makes you feel—albeit temporarily—that all is well.)

So why, you may wonder, are some people able to have cake or fried chicken without going off the deep end and overweight people aren't? Because many people have fewer dopamine receptors and are therefore more apt to crave foods that will increase dopamine. It's like the brain says, *"Ding ding ding!* We found a source of joy; go get more because we're running low!" And the brain communicates that by way of intense craving.

Once we ingest the fatty or sweet food, our bodies say, "Ahhhh," by releasing opiate-like substances into our bloodstream. It's like being hooked up to morphine . . . it's that feeling of being "comfortably numb." The problem is that, just like with drugs, we develop a tolerance and need more and more to get to that pleasant place. We eat larger and larger amounts of food, longing to feel that "sweet spot" of normal (part of the process is that when we aren't eating that stuff, we feel off-kilter; we're agitated, anxious, and depressed). If we can't get the food we want (and very large quantities of it), we go into withdrawal. If you've ever seen anyone detoxing from alcohol or drugs, you know it ain't pretty. Same with telling someone craving the feel-good of dopamine that she can't have her cheeseburger and apple pie, or to eat smaller portions. Having steamed vegetables and a bowl of beans or smaller portions simply isn't going to cut it.

And here's the kicker: the food industry panders to these cravings shamelessly, especially the fast-food industry. They want you to eat more food—cheap food. It's how they make money. They are in the business of selling products. So what makes you eat more of something? Fat and sugar! They exploit these natural cravings by adding into their products lots of fat and sugar, which just explodes the taste buds. You go crazy for that super rich, delicious taste, and it's very, very difficult to step away and be satisfied by healthy foods (sans the sugar and extra fat).

That's why today I want you to clean out your pantry and fridge of any junky foods that tempt you. Just get rid of them. You know what they are. Throw them out (or give them away) now.

That goes for all the food you know you can't stop eating once you start. For me, that would be chips. I simply cannot have just a few—especially barbecue-flavored ones. Same goes for chocolate chip cookies (oatmeal cookies could sit in my pantry forever), ice cream sandwiches, tapioca pudding, or any kind of cake. I could go on, really, but you get the drift. Make your house a safe zone, so that you have less ease and opportunity to eat the unhealthy stuff.

Whatever foods turn you into a zombie, no matter how much you swear you will only have "one more" or "just a bite"—toss 'em. After all, who ever has just one Oreo cookie, really? Who eats "just a few" chips? Who drinks half a soda? Just don't tempt yourself. Simple as that.

Then replace—or crowd out—that old habit. Fill the void with a healthier choice. Something chosen from the list of snacks or recipes at the back of this book. If you don't fill up that space with something delicious and non-addictive, you will likely feel deprived and fall back to your old poison. Especially at the beginning of this process, it's important to send yourself a message that your food choices remain abundant and fulfilling. For me, I swapped out ice cream and cake for some homemade rice pudding (suggestion in What to Eat Section); instead of chips I opted for tamari roasted almonds or bittersweet chocolate with goji berries. You're not deleting, you're upgrading!

Allow me, now, to apply the wisdom they use in AA for alcoholics (or drug addicts or debtors): Just for today, skip the (fill in the blank with your biggest tempter). Don't think about tomorrow or

Don't think about tomorrow or next year or the fact that you'd be so sad if you could never have it again. Just deal with today.

next year or the fact that you'd be so sad if you could never have it again. Just deal with today. Tell yourself this: "Just for today, I'm going to go without my poison." And make it easy on yourself by not even having the food around. (You might want to check out the 12-step program Overeaters Anonymous. It's free and there is one in just about every major town. You can also get their literature online at www.oa.org.

You'll probably have to enlist your family's help, especially if they are not joining you in the Lean. It's really important that you ask and that they respect your request for understanding.

And remember: Keep your eye on the prize, and keep trading up to healthier ways.

So, what are you going to do today?

- ✓ Drink lots of water.
- ✓ Eat a hearty breakfast.
- ✓ Eat an apple.
- ✓ Clean out the cupboards, and just for today, say no to your poison.

DAY 5.

Go a Little Nuts

AFTER YESTERDAY, YOU'RE GOING TO LIKE TODAY'S TWEAK. FOR YOUR midmorning snack, have a small fistful of raw, unsalted nuts or seeds. That's all there is to it.

I hope you didn't throw away (or give away) all your nuts in yesterday's cupboard purge. I know. Nuts aren't usually at the top of the dieter's "diet foods" list. And for some of you eating just one handful will be a challenge. But let me surprise you here. A body of research shows that eating nuts in moderation actually helps you lose weight. Here's the skinny . . .

Yes, nuts are packed with calories, but they are also packed with nutrition. And they fill you up, thereby "crowding out" room in your belly for high-calorie, nutrient-poor foods.

There have been nineteen clinical trials done to date on nuts and weight. In some cases, researchers added entire handfuls of nuts to people's daily diet. In two studies people did actually gain a few pounds, but in fourteen of the studies there was no significant weight change reported, and in the remaining three people actually lost weight! How is that even possible?

Let's look more closely at the research. These were clinical trials in which people were given nuts to eat for just a few weeks or months. But what about long term? Maybe in the short run nuts don't lead to weight gain, but what about years of eating nuts? Well, that's been looked at six different ways, in studies lasting from one year to eight years—including the now-famous Harvard Nurses' Health Study. One found no significant change, the other five out of six measures found *significantly less* weight gain, risk of being overweight, obesity, and abdominal obesity.

Yes, but what about *loss,* you may be asking. Well, trust me, when you are subbing nuts for chips or cheese or candy, you are breaking the cycle of snacking on highly addictive and fattening foods, and just by avoiding those old bad habits you will lose weight. If you don't eat chips or cheese or candy, you don't need nuts, per se; you may not need this tweak. But it's a huge step in the right direction if you're crowding out the bad for the healthy. Read on for the science, because there's even more to be said about metabolism and weight loss.

How is it possible that 90 percent of studies ever done on nuts and weight gain showed at the very least no weight gain? Where did the nut calories go? Doesn't that violate some pesky law of the physical universe that states that energy can neither be created nor destroyed? Calories don't just disappear.

One theory offered to the mystery of the missing calories has been called the "pistachio principle": Maybe nuts are just such a pain to eat that we don't end up eating as many. "For example," wrote a pair of researchers in a 2010 review, "in-shell pistachios slow the rate of consumption because of increased preparation time, and this may permit greater metabolic feedback during the ingestive event that augments satiety with the potential to reduce the energy content of the eating event." Meaning, nuts slow you down so your brain has time to think, *Hey, I'm eating—I better not eat too much!*

Okay, but what about pre-shelled nuts? Well, you still have to chew them. A study out of Japan suggests that "increasing dietary hardness [meaning difficulty of chewing] was associated with lower waist circumference." Your jaws burn some calories getting some exercise!

I mean, what if all you had to eat was raw cabbage all day? True, cabbage doesn't have many calories to begin with, but the tedium of chewing would presumably cause you to eat even less.

Then there's the "fecal excretion theory." A good portion of the cell walls of almonds, for example, remain intact in the GI tract throughout digestion, so even though nuts are high in calories, you may not absorb those calories because they stay behind. To test both these theories scientists would only need to compare weight gain from nuts to weight gain from nut butters.

Last year people studying the effects of peanut processing on body weight put both the pistachio principle and the fecal excretion theory to the test. Researchers said to themselves, let's feed a bunch of people a half cup of peanuts a day for a month, and another group the same amount of nuts but ground into peanut butter. So a half cup of peanuts, whole versus in peanut butter form.

This half cup was *added* to whatever each person was already eating in her regular diet, so calorie-wise, at the end of that month we'd expect to see some weight *gain.*

Well, as we saw before, in the whole nut peanut group that just didn't happen. The big question, though, is what happened to the peanut butter group? Not a lot of shelling or chewing going on there, and the cell walls of the peanuts were ground up, all the oil released, and made available for absorption. And they didn't go extra chunky; this was smooth peanut butter. If the lack of weight gain from nuts is due to all that chewing or fecal fat loss, then we'd expect that the peanut group would not pile on the pounds and the peanut butter group definitely would. But . . . they didn't.

Neither group gained the expected weight.

The plot thickens.

Maybe the reason why 90 percent of the relevant studies show no weight gain from nut consumption is that nuts are so satisfying, so satiating, so appetite suppressing that throughout the rest of the day—totally unconsciously, you just eat less.

Maybe adding 200 calories worth of nuts to your daily diet so satisfies you that you end up *not* eating 250 calories, or more, of something else! That could explain how you can remain in energy balance by adding a calorically dense food like nuts to your daily diet, and it might explain why in a few of the nut studies people actually *lost* weight.

Last year they tested walnuts. "It has been proposed, mainly on the basis of observational studies, that nuts may provide superior satiation, [and] may lead to reduced calorie consumption, but evidence from randomized, interventional studies is lacking," the scientists wrote. Until now.

They double-blinded the study by disguising the walnuts in a smoothie. "The walnut-containing liquid meal contained walnuts, frozen mango, frozen strawberries, banana, frozen berries, and pineapple juice." Sounds good.

The comparison smoothie had all the fruits and flavors but no nuts, just walnut flavoring. In fact the drinks rated as identical in taste in blind taste tests. And they were made with the exact same number of calories, so both groups should have felt equally satiated. But that's not what happened.

After a few days on the walnut-flavored, no-nut smoothie, people just felt something was missing. But the people who had the real walnut smoothies went on to eat a smaller lunch. The presence of the nuts in their smoothie resulted in decreased daily caloric consumption.

Yes, when we eat nuts we might lose some fat in our feces and have our appetite suppressed, but studies suggest that this accounts for just about 70 percent of the disappeared calories in nuts. Unless all the calories are accounted for we should still see weight gain after nut consumption, especially in the long term, but that's not what the studies showed.

So what happens to the last 30 percent?

Nuts appear to boost our metabolism, meaning when we eat nuts we burn more of our own fat to compensate. And indeed a new study showed that those on the control diet (without the walnuts) were burning about 20 grams of fat a day within their bodies. Not bad. That's like burning off 5 pats of butter.

Nuts appear to boost our metabolism, meaning when we eat nuts we burn more of our own fat to compensate.

But the walnut group, eating the same number of calories, the same amount of fat, same everything, burned more like 31 grams of fat a day—7 or 8 pats of butter. Not too shabby (or shall we say flabby)!

How do nuts do that? How do nuts boost fat burning within the body?

A 2010 paper out of Texas A&M University suggests that it may be the arginine content of nuts. How does arginine get the job done? They're not sure: "The underlying mechanisms are likely complex at molecular, cellular, and whole-body levels," they wrote—in other words, they have no clue. But they report some evidence that arginine may stimulate mitochondrial biogenesis—the creation of more furnaces per cell—and brown adipose tissue development, which is what your body uses to generate body heat: building more cellular furnaces and converting more of your fat into heat. Either way, these researchers expect arginine to play an important role in fighting the current global obesity epidemic.

Well, then, where in the diet do you find arginine? I'll give you a hint. According to the Centers for Disease Control, 77 million Americans aren't getting enough of it. So you know the top few sources have to be healthy foods, and indeed, here's the list of the top 15 food sources of arginine you'd likely find in a typical store, beginning with the richest source:

1. Soy protein isolate (6.7 grams per 100 grams), used in meat-free burgers and hot dogs
2. Pumpkin seeds (5.4 grams per 100 grams)
3. Squash seeds (5.4 grams per 100 grams)
4. Watermelon seeds (4.9 grams per 100 grams)—isn't that crazy? Not as crazy as . . .

5. Fried pork rinds (4.8 grams per 100 grams)—I'm not kidding.
6. Barbecue-flavored pork rinds (4.5 grams per 100 grams). It must concentrate in the skin.
7. Sesame seeds (3.3 grams per 100 grams)
8. Peanuts (3.25 grams per 100 grams)
9. Soybeans (3.15 grams per 100 grams)
10. Peanut butter (2.7 grams per 100 grams)
11. Tahini (2.68 grams per 100 grams)
12. Almonds (2.5 grams per 100 grams)
13. Pine nuts (2.4 grams per 100 grams)
14. Fava beans (2.4 grams per 100 grams)
15. Sunflower seeds (2.4 grams per 100 grams)

So for arginine it looks like our best bets are soy, seeds, nuts, and beans. Snails and beluga whale meat both have a lot, but the first non–pork rind animal food you could find in a typical store, according to the USDA database, clocks in at number 95: bacon.

What accounts for the thermogenic effect of nuts, their purported ability to boost metabolism so much that a person could potentially burn more fat just sitting around or sleeping?

The Texas A&M folks thought it was the arginine, but researchers at Purdue, in a study funded by Welch's entitled "The Effects of Concord Grape Juice on Appetite, Diet and Body Weight," produced evidence that it may be a phytonutrient effect. Just as nuts are calorically dense yet don't seem to cause weight gain, Welch's was keeping its fingers crossed that the same would be found for purple grape juice.

The researchers had people guzzle down two cups of grape juice a day for three months. Now, please understand, Welch's grape juice has more sugar than Coca-Cola. Two cups of purple grape juice contains the equivalent of 20 spoonfuls of sugar! The control group was basically given grape Kool-Aid: a "substitute grape drink," exact same number of calories, exact same amount of sugar, just without any detectable phytonutrients.

At two cups a day these folks were drinking in nearly 300 extra calories a day, surely after three months they must have gained a couple of pounds.

What do you think they found?

The grape-flavored sugar water group did indeed gain a significant amount of weight—how could they not with all that extra sugar in their diet? But the grape juice people didn't. In fact (are you ready for this?) their waist circumference shrank!

That's right. The group drinking two cups of grape juice a day for three months appeared to burn away significantly more tummy fat. Which would tend to support the theory put forth by the nut and green tea people, that flavonoid phytonutrients are capable of "increasing thermogenesis and fat oxidation." If true, that's just one more reason to eat nuts, drink green tea (we'll get to that on Day 9), and eat Concord grapes. (Please *eat* the grapes, though; don't drink them. It's too easy to drink up too much sugar and too many calories—in excess of what's healthy.)

In conclusion, the hard-to-crack nut of a mystery appears to have been solved: of all the calories you eat in nuts, 70 percent of them apparently disappear through dietary compensation mechanisms, 10 percent are flushed away, and 20 percent may be lost because of increased fat burn, leaving us with no calories to pack on any pounds; just a whopping load of nutrition and an appetite quelled.

So, what are you going to do today?

- ✓ Drink lots of water.
- ✓ Eat a hearty breakfast.
- ✓ Eat an apple.
- ✓ Just for today, say no to your poison.
- ✓ Go a little nuts.*

---

*If you have advanced heart disease, you may want to skip the nuts. You can read more on this in Dr. Caldwell Esselstyn's book Prevent and Reverse Heart Disease.

DAY 6.

Trade Your Milk and Butter for Plant-Based Versions

TODAY WE'RE GOING TO SWITCH UP MILK AND BUTTER FOR THEIR nondairy counterparts. And I'm going to point you to the yummiest ones.

Why this switch? Well, for starters, a lot of milk has added hormones in it—and these additives are no good for our waistlines. In fact, they're not good for the cows that produce the milk, let alone the humans who drink it! These hormones are injected into cows to make them produce more milk (which creates more profit). But even organic, grass-fed, and chemical-free milk is full of naturally occurring cow hormones that aren't necessarily good for people, whether the milk is whole, 2 percent, or skim.

Think of how milk happens: it's created by a lactating cow in order to feed her little calf so it will get really big, really quickly. By nature's brilliant design, this milk contains naturally occurring growth hormones in order to make a little one grow.

But we don't want to be fat, docile, and slow like cows. No sir; we want to be slim and quick on our feet. By the time we are in kindergarten, we're not drinking our mama's milk to make us bigger anymore, and we definitely don't need it from a cow whose milk is designed to put a hefty 1,000 pounds on her baby!

Cow's milk is the perfect nutrition for building a calf into a cow, but definitely not for a human—especially a human who would like to be slim. And to go even further, casein—the main protein in milk—is serious trouble for the human body. Casein is good for a nursing calf, because it helps her grow fast, and it's designed by nature to keep her bonded to mama. But when humans take in casein from the cow . . . oh, not good.

The casein in dairy is downright addictive. During the process of dairy digestion, the casein breaks apart into a host of opioids called casomorphins. Note the "morphin(e)" in there? Well, sure enough, when you ingest dairy, you get sort of addicted, as you might to morphine. Why so? Because nature designed cow's milk to have a drug-like effect on the calf's brain, to ensure that the little one stays bonded to the mom. It's nature's way of making sure the little one continues to get all the nutrients he or she needs. And by the way, just as opiates tend to be constipating, so can dairy products constipate you (especially cheese). So just know it's not for nothing that people say they are addicted to dairy; there's a reason! But that's why we are switching you to something better in such a way that you'll hardly miss a beat.

Let's get back to the nutritional issues. Might I mention that most of the fat in milk is saturated butterfat, which clogs your arteries and is bad for your heart? And according to T. Colin Campbell, professor emeritus of nutritional biochemistry at Cornell University and author of the groundbreaking book *The China Study*, that casein we were just talking about actually promotes *cancer*. In fact, he says casein is one of the most significant cancer promoters ever discovered. In layperson's terms: milk protein can fertilize cancer cells. (You can read more on this in my book *Veganist.*)

And besides all that, so many of us—80 percent of African Americans, 90 percent of Asian Americans, 60 percent of Hispanics, and many Caucasians are, to some degree, lactose intolerant, meaning drinking animal milk or eating products made from animal milk can cause us gas, pain, diarrhea, and other health problems.

(Lactose-free milk might help the lactose intolerance, but it still has casein in it.)

Trade your milk for nondairy versions and your stomach is likely to settle down real quickly. Not only that, the pounds will drop, too.

Putting the problem of casein aside for a moment, let's talk about skim milk.

> **A 2011 Harvard study of 12,829 children showed that skim milk may make you *fatter* than whole milk. The reason? Milk sugar.**

In a fascinating twist on expectation, a 2011 Harvard study of 12,829 children showed that skim milk may make you *fatter* than whole milk. That wouldn't surprise farmers; when they want to fatten up a pig, they feed it skim milk.

The reason? Milk sugar.

When you remove the fat from milk, what's left is lactose—milk sugar. The end product is an unbalanced, sugary-like drink that leads to weight gain.

So skip the nonfat and low-fat stuff and go for a yummy nondairy milk instead—preferably one that is unsweetened (although there are some nondairy milks that are sweetened with stevia; more on stevia in a couple of days).

I prefer the unsweetened nondairy milks so I can sweeten them, if I need to, to my own taste. Usually all it takes is a smidge of agave or stevia, but it's always better to see how much sugary stuff you're using and try to cool it wherever possible.

These days there are so many wonderful milk alternatives. You can find soy, almond, rice, hemp, or coconut milk just about anywhere, even at your favorite coffee place.

My half-sister, Kathy, a self-identified "creature of habit," loves Starbucks. She says, "One of my guilty pleasures is Starbucks. Now, instead of getting my drink with regular milk, I just get it with soy milk. Which they all carry. It's just no big deal." (Did I mention that she lost 30 pounds in less than 6 months?)

When you first taste nondairy milk you may not like it quite as much as cow's milk, but I assure you that you will come to love it after a very short time. (Remember, cow's milk is physiologically addictive, so once it's out of your system, you'll be A-OK. Just make the switch today, and after a short bit, you won't miss it at *all*.) A few years after I'd given up cow's milk I accidentally had a latte with the cow stuff, and it tasted gamey and thick. Any fond old thoughts I harbored about the milk I grew up with were gone for good.

Cow's milk is physiologically addictive, so once it's out of your system, you'll be A-OK. Just make the switch today, and after a short bit, you won't miss it at *all*.

Seriously, you will come to love the nonanimal versions of milk! You can heat it up and pour it over your breakfast grains (I alternate between soy, rice, almond, and hemp), add it to your tea or coffee, cook with it just like you would milk (I make some fierce mashed sweet potatoes using soy milk), or use it in a smoothie.

You'll feel extra good about making this switch when I tell you that the USDA and the Department of Health and Human Services just released their *Dietary Guidelines for Americans* in January 2011, in which they provide advice on how good dietary habits can promote health and reduce risk for major chronic diseases. The guidelines emphasize a plant-based diet! Most people think that plant-based foods are just fruits and vegetables, but they include whole grains, nuts, legumes, and soy foods like soy milk, almond milk, and coconut milk.

Plant-based foods are associated with lower rates of heart disease, stroke, and diabetes because they tend to be high in nutrients and low in calories and saturated fat. Research has also shown that plant-based foods can help reduce the risk of chronic disease. For example, most plant-based foods are much lower in saturated fat than animal foods, making them a better choice for maintaining heart health. Also, since plant-based foods contain no cholesterol, using

---

Since plant-based foods contain no cholesterol, using them to replace animal foods can be an effective way to lower overall cholesterol intake.

---

them to replace animal foods can be an effective way to lower overall cholesterol intake.

One reader, a man named Mac, told me he'd always had high cholesterol—over 300!—but after changing his diet for just four weeks he went in for a cholesterol check and was astonished at the results:

Well, it was 196—the lowest it had EVER been in the 30+ years I'd been testing. To top it off I'd lost almost 30 pounds in less than four weeks—without any increase in physical activity.

The simple switch away from animal foods had an amazing—and amazingly fast—effect on Mac's health. And he'd only just begun!

But back to milk. A reader named Yvonne wrote to me about switching her milks:

The biggest thing for me was finding a new milk. I just can't live without cereal! So I tried rice milk and it was too sweet and watery. I tried almond and didn't love it either. I landed on soy and fell in love. I think it's hardest when you are first transitioning, because you are used to how "regular milk" tastes, and "regular cheese." So the initial switch was tricky because I wanted the substitute products to taste like the things I was used to. I didn't like the rice cheese, but I also ate a slice on its own. So then I tried hiding it in a wrap and it was okay . . . In hindsight I would put some distance between eating the "old" products and trying the new versions. Nondairy cheese and ice cream are just not going to taste the exact same. But in time I discovered they are delicious! It is just different. But going in expecting to not notice the difference was silly.

One "nutrient of concern" noted by the new *Dietary Guidelines* is calcium. Since consumers do not get enough of this vital nutrient, many makers of soy, almond, and coconut milks have recently increased the calcium level in their products to equal that of conventional dairy milk, or they even surpass it by 50 percent! Fifty percent more calcium than milk: well, you can't beat that!

Just remember when you hear arguments in favor of dairy—"but you need milk for strong bones"—that the National Dairy Council is all about supporting and perpetuating a big, profitable industry, and they spend a lot of money coming up with marketing campaigns and sponsoring studies to support their claims.

Just use your head and question their motives, and think on the fact that for thousands of years the Chinese never used milk and they were slim and healthy, with very low cholesterol. It's only been recently, since the Western way of eating meat and dairy has been introduced, that the Chinese have started getting fatter and sicker.

Butter

Now to everyone's favorite fat: butter. Butter makes everything taste better. Okay, agreed. But butter is nearly all fat—much of it saturated fat—and it's calorie dense. One tablespoon of butter has 102 calories. Compare that to hummus, which has only 25 calories for the same tablespoon. If you're looking for a spread for your toast or cracker, try using hummus or some other bean spread. You can even smear a little avocado where you would have used butter. If you are sautéing something, try using a little spray olive oil, and when I say a little, I mean like a super-quick spritz.

And if you consider the taste of butter an absolute must-have every once in a while, try Earth Balance buttery spread. It's delicious and substitutes perfectly anywhere you'd use butter.

If you've heard nasty things about margarine—and they're likely true—don't worry: Earth Balance is not margarine.

Here's the unhealthy scoop about butter and margarine. Aside from cholesterol, the problem with butter is saturated fat. Eating too much saturated fat increases "bad" cholesterol, and even though it also raises "good" cholesterol, it's not enough to justify eating it. Since saturated fat increases the risk of heart disease, the amount recommended is between 10–15 grams. One little pat of butter has over 7 grams!

Margarine is different, but no better. It has trans fats, which have been shown to increase "bad" cholesterol while tending to lower "good" cholesterol. And it makes our blood platelets stickier, which increases heart attack risk. One tablespoon of stick margarine packs 3 grams of transfat and 2 grams of saturated fat. Nunja good!

The good news: Earth Balance tastes pretty much exactly like the butter you grew up loving. It's made from expeller-pressed oils and has been shown to support healthy cholesterol; it's free of trans fats and hydrogenated oil, and it's rich in the highly beneficial omega-3 fatty acids (more on omega-3s on Day 11). It does have a similar calorie count to butter, though, so you want to use it sparingly.

Taste around, try different brands, find the nut milks or soy milks that you like best. Keep a stick or tub of Earth Balance on hand for special occasions. In short order, you won't miss a thing, and you'll surely need to buy a new (smaller) belt.

So, what are you going to do today?

✓ Drink lots of water.
✓ Eat a hearty breakfast.
✓ Eat an apple.
✓ Just for today, say no to your poison.
✓ Go a little nuts.
✓ Trade up the milk and butter.

DAY 7.

Put a Little Flax on It

TODAY'S LEAN WILL TAKE JUST A MOMENT OR TWO AND YIELD SIGNIFI-cant rewards. All I want you to do is add in two tablespoons of ground flaxseed somewhere in your day. Add them to any foods you like (as long as they end up in your mouth). Flax has a sweet, nutty flavor, so it goes down easily!

You can sprinkle ground flax over your breakfast rice or oat-meal, add it to a smoothie, mix it into your salad, or stir it into a soup or veggie stew or casserole. There are as many uses for ground flax as your imagination will allow. And it is a huge boost to any weight loss plan.

> **Extra Lean:** Enjoy soups more often because they take longer to eat and therefore slow you down. You can hardly wolf down a piping hot bowl of lentil and onion soup; it takes time to blow off the steam and let it cool down in your mouth!

Why?

It's bulk, baby! Fabulous fiber yet again. You'd have to look high and low to get a food that's this high in fiber, both soluble and insoluble. Soluble fiber just means that it absorbs water, expands and forms a gel-like substance, which takes up more room in your stomach and delays the time it takes for food to digest. To be more precise, the fiber slows down the passage of food across the valve that sends signals from the small intestines to the large intestines. Your body then receives appetite suppressing signals that tell you you're full. See, your body is actually being reprogrammed! And because everything is slowed down, your blood sugar remains stable and you *stay* feeling full or sated for longer.

Insoluble fiber is more like what your parents called "roughage"; it doesn't really break down, but it pushes things through the digestive system. One ounce of flaxseed provides 32 percent of your daily dose of fiber, so it's an excellent assurance that you'll eat fewer calories while feeling more energetic throughout the day. It's yet another way to crowd out the hungry beast! But that's not all that flax has to offer.

Flaxseeds are low in carbs, high in most of the B vitamins, and are an excellent source of omega-3 fatty acids and a good source of omega 6. Flax is also the most concentrated dietary source of lignans, which the good bacteria in our gut turn into the powerful cancer-fighting compounds that not only significantly lower breast cancer risk in the first place but may double the survival rates of breast cancer patients. The Long Island Breast Cancer Study Project estimated that the quantity of lignans women average daily from their entire diet is about 6 milligrams. That's how many lignans are found in just a single teaspoon of flaxseeds. So adding even just a teaspoon of

> **Flaxseeds are low in carbs, high in most of the B vitamins, and are an excellent source of omega-3 fatty acids.**

> **Flax is also the most concentrated dietary source of lignans, which the good bacteria in our gut turn into powerful cancer-fighting compounds.**

ground flaxseeds to your diet may double your entire intake for the day.

Flaxseeds have also been shown to lower bad cholesterol levels, improve blood pressure, control hot flashes in women, and work just as well as the leading drug for enlarged prostate symptoms in men—but with only good side effects. Flax was often used to heal digestive troubles in the times of the Roman Empire, and Hippocrates (the father of medicine) apparently used it as one of his valued "medicines." Mahatma Gandhi famously said, "Wherever flaxseed becomes a regular food item among the people, there will be better health."

You can buy flaxseeds already ground, and they can last for 6 weeks in the fridge in an airtight container. Or you can buy them whole and grind them yourself—I always keep a bag of flaxseeds in my fridge, and I grind up about 6 tablespoons (three days' worth) at a time in a coffee grinder that I don't use for coffee (lest the taste cross over). (If they aren't ground, the seeds will pass through your system whole, and you won't get all the nutritional benefits from them.)

You can take your 2 tablespoons all at once, or split up your dose throughout the day, making each meal more fulfilling and guarding you against the munchies. Easy peasy, short and sweet!

So, what are you going to do today?

✓ Drink lots of water.
✓ Eat a hearty breakfast.
✓ Eat an apple.
✓ Just for today, say no to your poison.
✓ Go a little nuts.
✓ Trade up the milk and butter.
✓ Put a little flax on it.

DAY 8.

Do a Deep Dive for Five

LOOK AT YOU! YOU'VE BEEN AT THE LEAN FOR A FULL WEEK. CON-gratulations. You've been crowding out the bad stuff and filling yourself up with delicious, highly nutritious foods and trying new milks and figuring out just how easy leaning really is.

Now it's time to get a little introspective. What has stopped you from reaching your weight loss goals before? And why do you tend to eat more calories than you should, even though you know you won't like the long-term outcome of being overweight?

As you read on Day 3, sugary and fatty foods trigger brain chemicals that cause you to crave them; that's one reason you eat more than you should. You've also read that if you don't get the right nutrients and fiber, your body will send you out for more food because it's still not satisfied with what you've given it.

Today, we're going to dig around and find out what feelings or issues you are avoiding or glossing over by *trance eating*—a term I use to describe the eating we do to distract ourselves from uncomfortable thoughts and emotions. Because, after all, when we eat without thinking, when we're totally focused on the tastes and textures and guilt and shame and craving, we are acting in a trance. When we are in a food trance—whether we're working through a box of cookies or a whole pizza pie—everything else gets pushed to the side. No worrying about anything else; it's all about the food. We've gone unconscious.

The word *unconscious* refers to an emotional activity that is below our level of awareness. The feelings we can deal with and understand are conscious. For instance, you might be conscious that you are angry with your boss. You can deal with that anger by talking with the human relations department or looking for another job. That's the sort of emotion that's the tip of the iceberg—you see it, it's understandable, and you can navigate it. But in another instance, you might *not* be conscious of the anger you have at your child or your spouse because this person takes up so much of your time and energy, and you can't just do what you really want to do. That feeling falls into the unconscious category—you don't even know you're angry. It's the underbelly of the iceberg.

The unconscious holds the stuff that is scary and threatening ("What the hell am I supposed to do if I am angry at my kid? I can't just leave . . ."). So it gets pushed down, repressed. Traumatic memories, such as childhood emotional or sexual abuse, also may fall into the unconscious. We don't want to think of the things that we can't understand or do anything about. It's a survival instinct to push them down and away. But here's the thing: to know what's in the unconscious is extremely important, because what goes on in there may very well be responsible for your trance eating and weight problems. As the old adage goes, "If you bring forth what is within you, what is within you will save you. If you do not bring forth what is within you, what is within you will kill you." Or make you fat.

Today I want you to take a few moments to get to know yourself a little better, to understand what's going on inside of you and make peace with it. Because if you bring to the surface some of that which is unconscious, you might no longer need the food compulsion to keep you distracted. I don't want you to numb out. I don't want you to spend your life blocking things from your awareness or escaping into food. I want you to be free, and freedom requires that you go in and take a look around at your psyche. And having taken a look around, make some peace. You might even begin to make a few subtle, gentle shifts in your life.

Oh, by the way, you can do this in *five minutes,* so no excuses. I'm not suggesting deep therapy (although do go if you have the time and money; there's no one who wouldn't benefit from a little psychological guidance). I'm just suggesting that you give yourself five little minutes a day to devote to your personal growth and introspection. The more you know and accept yourself, the less you need to disappear behind the thick layers of unhealthy eating. Here's what you do.

Start off by being still. Sit down where you won't be bothered so that you can give yourself your full attention, or take a walk someplace by yourself. By being quiet, you'll be able to listen for cues from your inner knowingness. Your ideas and intuitions can come to the surface when you pull yourself away from the daily routine, if even just for a few minutes. Try to drop your attention beneath the surface of what you show the world and into the real you. No judgment allowed in the Deep Dive for Five, just observation.

Ask yourself, "What am I feeling now?" "What do I need to look at?" Try to locate what is really going on inside of you. All too often, we try to put forward what we think others want to see in us. We try and act cool or laid-back; we try to appear carefree or happy, when in fact we might very well be angry or sad. We mask our truth because sometimes our truth doesn't seem to fit in with others and it makes them uncomfortable; sometimes people outright reject us for feeling the way we feel.

Feelings are funny; they won't go away even if we tell them to. They won't change to suit our desire to be different. They will just hang out in the basement of our psyche and come out in inappropriate and destructive ways, like trance eating. You can short-circuit trance eating, though, by getting still and listening to the insights that bubble up. Sometimes those insights float into your awareness through thoughts, and sometimes they are in the body itself.

When feelings are overridden by shame or doubt, they often get pressed down into our cells, into our very physical being. They become repressed. What the mind tries to ignore, the body often belies by aches, pains, or odd sensations. Our bodies will give us hints at what we should know or be careful of, even if we may not be consciously aware of what the truth is, so check in with your body to see if it's trying to tell you something.

For instance, you may feel nauseated at the thought of someone, while "on paper" they seem to be perfectly nice. Your mind tells you that you should like them and invite them in, but your body says that something is not right. You might feel a flush of anxiety, or perhaps get a splitting headache right before having to visit a certain person. These are things to honor and pay attention to. Even if it's inconvenient to get someone out of your life, or if it will upset the apple cart, it's worthwhile at least considering what your gut is telling you.

If you get quiet and focus on whatever you are feeling in your physical being, you will begin to notice which emotions are lurking just beneath the surface. Sometimes a backache or a neck spasm is a distraction from feelings of anxiety or rage, and in the same way, intense food cravings are also a distraction. The tricky mind figures that if we focus on physical pain or food cravings and eating compulsions, we won't have to deal with emotional discomfort.

But consider this: just as you can breathe into a pain and it will connect to the unconscious emotion likely attached to it, so can you breathe into food issues. Things are quite often deeper than they appear to be.

Again, I'm not asking you to act on anything, or even to change something. I'm just asking you to apply some mindfulness to whatever comes up. So if you are about to meet with someone and you get a gnawing, uncomfortable feeling in your belly, you might stop and ask yourself, "What is really going on? What is my body trying to tell me?" In that same vein, if you have the intense desire to go to Baskin-Robbins or order out for Domino's, you might stop and ask yourself, "What is this craving trying to cover up? What am I trying to distract myself from?" Then take a few deep breaths while you listen and intuit the wisdom, and see if it is followed by some inner guidance. Say to yourself the following:

Ask yourself, "What is this craving trying to cover up? What am I trying to distract myself from?"

> *I am listening. I'm okay with whatever feelings and thoughts are beneath the surface.*

And then send yourself some love and compassion, knowing that being aware of the truth will always lead to the next right step, if a step is needed at all. Remember, optimal health—and healthy weight is part of that—is achieved through the integration of body, mind, and soul. A vital part of the weight loss process is discovering the roots of the emotional components, untangling them, and transforming them.

Keeping things locked up inside is stressful. And when we are chronically stressed, our bodies produce more of the hormone cortisol, which in excess causes us to gain weight, especially in the belly area. Stress also causes us to seek out fattening comfort foods. By doing the Deep Dive, you have essentially done a five-minute mindfulness meditation, and meditation is an excellent tool for weight loss. When you make peace with your thoughts and emotions during the Deep Dive, or whenever you meditate, you are less likely to use food as an emotional crutch. Many people overeat or eat unhealthy foods to fill voids within their lives; with this meditation, you will be filling the void and calming your inner chaos with your attention and breath. A daily meditation will help you to break the emotional eating cycle by making you more aware of your mental, emotional, and physical processes. You

A daily meditation will help you to break the emotional eating cycle.

will find that instead of automatically reaching for food, you will have the ability to make more conscious choices. The Deep Dive helps interrupt the mental dialogue that often leads to unhealthy eating, and you can ask yourself, "Is this really going to make me feel better?"

> **Extra Lean:** Think before you eat. Ask yourself if you are really, truly hungry. Perhaps you are thirsty instead? Or tired and need a rest? Or emotional and need a conversation with a good friend? Or anxious and would be better off taking a brisk walk. If you still want to snack, consider what you are putting in your body, and what the long-term results of feeding yourself a particular food are. Eat mindfully and slowly.

There's no need to drag this process out; just take a few minutes to check in and see how you are doing. Take your emotional temperature, and breathe in some peace. Set your watch or phone alarm so that you aren't worried about time, and let yourself sink in. Finish up with a quick visualization of yourself being content, healthy, and thriving.

So, what are you going to do today?

✓ Drink lots of water.
✓ Eat a hearty breakfast.
✓ Eat an apple.
✓ Just for today, say no to your poison.
✓ Go a little nuts.
✓ Trade up the milk and butter.
✓ Put a little flax on it.
✓ Do a deep dive for five.

DAY 9.

Switch Up Your Drinks

I GREW UP IN ATLANTA, GEORGIA—THE HOME OF COCA-COLA—AND let's just say that I took incredible pride in supporting the local economy! To me, Cokes and the like were manna from heaven. I loved that sweet and salty, syrupy taste as much as all my friends did, and nothing seemed as innocent and all-American as drinking down an ice cold soda after school.

But boy, one was never enough. Once you get that taste in your mouth, you want—need—more. And then more. And more still. I swear there should be a 12-step program for soda drinkers!

If you're not a soda drinker, you can breeze right through this tweak. But a full 1 out of 4 Americans does drink at least one soda per day, and that's serious trouble for the waistline. Typical big-brand colas are loaded with sugar and high fructose corn syrup (HFCS), so much so that it might be more accurate to think of them as liquid candy. And just like candy, typical sodas have zero nutritional value, are highly addictive, and put weight on you almost immediately. We'll talk more about how sugar and HFCS put on weight on Day 23, but for now let's just get you weaned off the stuff, and focus on bumping you up to a better habit.

Moving away from sugary sodas is one little thing you can do that will have you feeling better right away, and your weight will quickly reflect the shift.

Moving away from sugary sodas is one little thing you can do that will have you feeling better right away, and your weight will quickly reflect the shift.

If you are used to drinking something sparkling and sweet, I know it might be too much to ask of you to simply switch to water, so I won't. (This tweak, by the way, is not to replace drinking the 8 glasses of water a day. I want you to keep that up, too.) Instead, I'm going to ask you to upgrade to a drink that tastes almost as good as what you are used to but that doesn't have sugar or HFCS in it.

And while you're at it, I'd also like you to avoid the chemical sweeteners found in diet drinks because (a) they can cause digestive discomfort and bloating, and (b) some of those chemical sweeteners have been found to be cancer causing. You just don't need 'em.

You can simply squeeze a little lemon or lime, or add a little unsweetened fruit concentrate, into some sparkling water or club soda, and add a touch of stevia or agave to sweeten it.

To keep the price down, rather than buying bottles of club soda every week I invested in a home soda maker (the one I have is called SodaStream), which is great for making homemade colas out of your tap water. If you decide to use one of those, throw out the flavor packs it comes with, because they also have chemicals and sugar (and they don't taste very good either, in my humble opinion).

When I make my own soda, I usually add a little bit of pomegranate, cherry, or cranberry concentrate (you can find them in most grocery or health food stores, or order them online) to the sparkling water, and then sweeten to taste with a touch of liquid stevia. (I opt for stevia over agave, because with agave you are still going to get calories and a bit of an insulin response, although it's certainly much better than sugar or HFCS. More on all this later.)

You might also make yourself some thirst-quenching lemonade

with either fresh lemons or lemon concentrate, and sweeten to taste. As a regular, everyday beverage that is nice to drink with meals, try iced herbal tea. You can try different flavors like açaí berry (my favorite), lemon zinger, or cranberry zest. They are refreshing and have no calories, and will complement your dishes without overwhelming them with strong flavors.

Juice

Now I'll say a few words about juice, because I know it may seem like a healthy thing to indulge in. This should tell you something: if a diabetic begins to go into a coma because of plummeting blood sugar, he is advised to consume some orange or other fruit juice so that his body will be flooded with sugar and he'll snap out of it. It's *that* sweet, even without added sugar. So, if it's not one of the green juices we'll be talking about on Day 25, don't drink it.

Even though apple juice, orange juice, grapefruit juice, et cetera, are all made from delicious, healthy fruit, they are still loaded with naturally occurring sugar. It takes quite a few pieces of fruit to make up one glass of juice, so you are getting a lot of fruit sugar without the fiber to slow the absorption, and that just packs on pounds. (Fruit eaten whole is fine, just not fruit juice.)

If you are used to having juice with breakfast, I know it will be hard to pull yourself off, but pull yourself you must! Have some iced tea instead, or some water with lemon or lime squeezed into it.

Booze

As for alcohol, keep it moderate (unless you suspect you are an addict, in which case you should skip it altogether). No more than one drink a day for women, and preferably only a few days a week, and two drinks for men. Curiously, alcohol itself does not raise your blood sugar level; it actually lowers it, by inhibiting the liver from releasing glycogen (carbohydrates stored in the liver and released for energy when you're between meals). Your liver treats the alcohol like a toxin and goes about the detoxification process, putting off releasing glycogen till it is complete. And since this is a slow process that means you can go without a steady release of glycogen for a long time, which can lead to hypoglycemia (low blood sugar). And we all know that low blood sugar makes you want to eat. A lot.

What does raise our blood sugar level when we drink alcohol are the carbohydrates contained in the drink, and that is what is turned into glucose in our body. Most alcoholic drinks have a high simple carbohydrate content (sugars from the grapes in wine, the malt in beer or scotch), and this will flood your system with glucose. Your pancreas releases insulin in order to handle the glucose at the same time that the liver is impaired by detoxification. What you can get is a fluctuating blood sugar level, with all its attendant problems (including insulin resistance). This is something to keep in mind, because healthy weight depends on stable blood sugar levels.

Healthy weight depends on stable blood sugar levels.

And of course something else to consider is that when you are drinking, your judgment tends to get wonky. Booze relaxes inhibitions, and thus you get more relaxed about what you eat. The part of us that is health conscious gets shunted aside and off you go to satisfy your munchies. Plus, there are psychological associations between certain drinks and foods, like beer and chips, or wine and cheese. Indulging in fattening foods just goes with the territory in a night of drinking. I know too many people who have put on some serious pounds just by eating "hangover food"; I have one friend who craved Big Macs and fries the morning after a few drinks, and after a year of indulging she'd put on a good 30 pounds. If you don't want to drink and everyone else is having cocktails, just put a splash of pomegranate juice into a martini glass with some ice-cold water and a lemon twist so that it looks festive, and you can sip on it slowly and not call attention to yourself.

Coffee

Discussing coffee's place in a healthy diet elicits very conflicted (and passionate!) opinions. I myself have had an on-again, off-again relationship with it. For years, coffee was blamed for everything from high blood pressure to decreased bone density and cognitive impairment. Newer research, however, indicates that there are some compelling reasons to enjoy coffee in moderation.

The words *coffee* and *caffeine* may seem synonymous, but the fact is that caffeine isn't the only compound in coffee; it also contains lots of antioxidants. When coffee is enjoyed in moderation (meaning about 3 cups a day for an average person) it may actually have measurable health *benefits*, including protective effects against diseases like Alzheimer's, type 2 diabetes, and even colon cancer. You can gain these benefits even if you drink decaf, although decaf coffee does contain small amounts of caffeine too.

Coffee drinkers may also reap some modest weight loss benefits as well. One fairly well-known benefit is coffee's appetite suppressant quality. As an appetite suppressant, it doesn't rank with dangerous substances like ephedrine, and it certainly shouldn't be relied on to take the place of food or other drinks but only as a bonus best used in conjunction with a healthy overall diet. If you're susceptible to heartburn or acid reflux, or just have a sensitive stomach, you may benefit from one of the lower-acid coffees like HealthWise or Folger's Simply Smooth.

Dietary thermogenic properties are another characteristic of coffee that can supplement weight loss. Thermogenesis is the body's production of heat as a result of the physiological processes of metabolism, and coffee is a mildly thermogenic beverage. What this means for moderate coffee drinkers is a slight increase in calories burned after drinking a cup of coffee—about 10 percent. Like coffee's modest appetite diminishing effect, the increase in fat burning doesn't last all day, and it isn't effective as a primary or sole method of shedding excess weight. But used within the context of a lifestyle incorporating an abundance of *other* small adjustments, coffee can be an ally.

Athletes know that coffee also functions as a performance booster. A 2009 *New York Times* article stated that numerous studies have led researchers to the consensus that a cup of coffee before a workout improves your performance and endurance during exercise. And in 2011, the *New York Times* again reported on the same effects, this time citing more recent research that came to the same conclusion: coffee can galvanize your workout. Just make sure not to overdo it and get *too* wired.

All these benefits are great, but what's the caveat with coffee? Usually it's in the empty calories that are added to it. Calories and fat in the form of milk, sugar, and creamer will quickly obliterate any weight loss benefit that you might otherwise get. Have you ever been asked—or asked yourself—if you'd "like a little coffee with your cream and sugar?" If so, these effortless refinements can make the transition to a healthier cup easy and painless:

• Substitute unsweetened almond, coconut, or soy milk for milk or cream. Try different varieties until you find one you like; virtually all will taste richer and more satisfying than any skim or fat-free dairy. Silk Soy creamer is my favorite for hot beverages, as the creamer is thicker than the regular nondairy milks and thus blends better. Only a tad is needed.

• Use stevia in place of sugar (again, refrain from using artificial sweeteners) and to sweeten the milk if needed.

You should also apply these changes to the coffee you drink on the go. A Starbucks single Grande (16-ounce) Caffè Mocha with 2 percent milk packs a whopping 330 calories and 33 grams of sugar. The "skinny" versions are no improvement, since the syrups used in these drinks contain artificial sweeteners similar to Splenda, otherwise known by its chemical name, sucralose. Splenda's tagline may be "made from sugar" but in reality it's a chemically altered *synthetic* sugar-*like* molecule that was manufactured in a lab. Instead, order the regular brewed coffee and ask for a shot of soy milk. I keep a few packs of stevia in my purse and in my car so I can add that as a sweetener if I'm at a place that only carries sugar and chemical sweeteners. And with a typical latte costing anywhere from $3 to $5 and a regular cup of coffee approaching $2, you won't just be saving calories but also money!

It's important to keep in mind, too, that taking periodic extended "coffee breaks" and allowing your body to relearn how to function without the stimulation may have health benefits, so I advise you not to become (or remain) dependent on the buzz. And don't forget that coffee is a diuretic, so be sure to drink extra water while you're on coffee so that you keep your body nice and hydrated.

Let me be clear here. Drinking coffee is certainly not mandatory; I'm only addressing it in case you are a coffee drinker and wondering if you can and should continue. If you feel heart palpitations or anxiety as a result of drinking coffee, stop. And you certainly don't need to start drinking coffee if you don't already.

Green Tea

A better option might be green tea, both for overall health and for weight loss. Some studies suggest that green tea can raise metabolism, which causes the body to burn more calories, probably because of phytochemicals in the tea called catechins. And not only do you get a revved up metabolism, but it seems that drinking green tea also activates a higher rate of fat oxidation, meaning that the body can better break down fats to be used as energy.

> **Drinking green tea activates a higher rate of fat oxidation, meaning that the body can better break down fats to be used as energy.**

One study fed 38 Japanese people the same diet, but one group drank tea. The people in that group consumed a bottle of tea containing 690 milligrams of catechin antioxidants per day. At the end of 12 weeks, their body fat mass, waist size, BMI, and body weight were significantly lower than in the group that did not get the green tea. The researchers concluded that the catechin antioxidants in green tea help to reduce body fat and control obesity.

In another small study, researchers assigned 10 men to receive either a dose of green tea extract plus caffeine, caffeine alone, or a placebo. When the men received the dose of green tea extract plus caffeine, they burned more calories than when they received just caffeine or a placebo, which would indicate that aside from caffeine, green tea has something in it that stimulates fat burning and thermogenesis (calories burned as heat during digestion).

Green tea has important antioxidants and compounds that help maintain good health, and there is evidence that it may help prevent heart disease, dementia, diabetes, cancer, and even extend our life span. One thing is absolutely sure, and that is that green tea is a refreshing drink without any calories and a healthy beverage to add in to the Lean plan.

So, what are you going to do today?

- ✓ Drink lots of water.
- ✓ Eat a hearty breakfast.
- ✓ Eat an apple.
- ✓ Just for today, say no to your poison.
- ✓ Go a little nuts.
- ✓ Trade up the milk and butter.
- ✓ Put a little flax on it.
- ✓ Do a deep dive for five.
- ✓ Switch up your drinks.

DAY 10.

Make Your Lunch without Animal Products

I IMAGINE IT HAS REGISTERED WITH YOU ALREADY, BUT IN CASE IT HASN'T, let me point it out. For over a week now you've been cutting back on animal products. I started you off with meatless breakfasts, and we've talked about going without animal milk, too. Today we're going to push it a little farther and have you go meatless for lunch, just to really nudge the process forward.

Meatless means no flesh from an animal, so that includes pork, lamb, beef, chicken, turkey, and fish. I know you probably rely on turkey and Swiss sandwiches or chicken salad or beef burritos. They're the lunches you grew up with and they may be the only foods available near your office, right? You might be wondering what the heck you're going to put on your plate if it's not meat or dairy. Please know that this is indeed a big lean, but the payoff is quite extraordinary in terms of your weight and your health—which of course are inextricably linked.

Remember the "revolutionary" promise I made to you with the subtitle of this book? Never let it be said that I make empty promises! Here's the thing: the word *revolution*, as defined in the dictionary, means "outside or beyond the established procedure, principles, etc." Well, the established diet of choice for the past few

> **The established diet of choice for the past few decades has been one full of animal protein and low on carbs, and if you look around, the population hasn't been getting any slimmer. No, in fact, we've become alarmingly obese.**

decades has been one full of animal protein and low on carbs, and if you look around, the population hasn't been getting any slimmer. No, in fact, we've become alarmingly obese. And if you've been swept up in this craze, or simply tried one or more of the popular diets touting success through eating anything that flies, swims, or walks, you've most likely not enjoyed great and lasting success in your weight loss endeavors.

And it's not at all your fault. The body does not want to do itself damage, but by eating that way, damage is indeed done. Read on.

Yes, you will probably lose weight on a high-protein, low-carb diet. But the weight loss comes partly from eating fewer calories because you are knocking out so much of what you normally would consume, and partly because these days eliminating carbohydrates means doing away with calorie-dense, highly processed foods (most of which contain HFCS). Of *course* you lose weight when you give up cookies and cakes and doughnuts, which erroneously get lumped together, even in "good" diets like Weight Watchers, with good carbs like those from brown rice and quinoa. But eating a high-protein, low-carb diet doesn't work long term. Not only that, it wreaks serious damage to your precious body.

Since we are on the subject of "revolution," I've pulled some incredibly informative quotes from Chapter Four of John Robbins's book, *The Food Revolution: How Your Diet Can Help Save Your Life and Our World,* which sum up why it's time to turn away from the way we've been dieting. Here's a sample of what Robbins reported:

As reported by *CBS HealthWatch by Medscape* in December 1999, Dr. James W. Anderson, professor of medicine and clinical nutrition at the University of Kentucky, said this about the Atkins diet:

On Atkins, "people lose weight, at least in the short term. . . . But this is absolutely the worst diet you could imagine for long-term obesity, heart disease, and some forms of cancer." Dr. Anderson noted in 1999 that there were 18 million diabetics in this country, and 55 million people with high blood pressure [Those numbers have greatly increased to date]. "They can have kidney problems—and high protein intake will bring them on faster," Anderson said. He explained that the diet is thrombogenic. "This means the fat will tend to form lipid particles in your blood after meals, which could lead to blood clots, meaning heart attack or stroke. We worry about this because many of the people who love these diets are men aged 40 to 50, who like their meat. They may be 5 years from their first heart attack." Anderson added that for 50 percent of men who suffer fatal heart attacks, the fatal attack is the first symptom. "They will never know what this diet is doing to them."

Here's the cornerstone claim of how the Atkins diet works: the body goes into something called ketosis, which is similar to what happens when someone is starving and the body begins to eat up muscle because of an imbalance in fat metabolism. The problem is that when ketosis goes on for too long, it causes serious kidney problems and an increased risk of heart disease, and for pregnant women it can cause abnormalities in the fetus or miscarriage. It can also be fatal for diabetics. The body ultimately can't sustain this diet, and people who try it nearly always quit and gain back all their weight and then some. In fact, studies show that most people gain back an average of 5 percent more than what they originally started with. So it's not only not working long term, but you are likely to actually gain more back than what you started with.

Give that smart body of yours credit for revolting and getting off this kind of crazy diet. It knows this diet is not good. So it prompts you to go back to some carbs, and before you know it, you are back to your old weight and more. (We need carbs, but if you are going back to refined carbs rather than wholesome, unrefined carbs, you get into trouble; but more on that later.)

A diet similar to Atkins is the Zone; but here is what the Center for Science in the Public Interest's nutrition director, Bonnie Liebman said about the Zone diet:

"[Barry] Sears' advice will probably help you lose weight . . . but only because you will be eating fewer calories . . . And to experts who have seen miracle diets come and go like hemlines, hair-dos, and celebrity romances, that's nothing new." Liebman said that like most fad diets, the Zone is based "on an eensy-weensy kernel of truth . . . blown way out of proportion by theory, not evidence."

Peter D'Adamo, author of *Eat Right for Your Type,* a "blood type" diet, maintains that if you are a type O (like me and about 40 percent of the population, according to the American Red Cross), you need to eat a lot of red meat in order to be healthy and slim. D'Adamo bases this on his theory that Cro-Magnon people, who lived 20,000 to 30,000 years ago, were type O and thrived mostly on meat and therefore anyone with type O blood is genetically equipped to eat meat, not grains.

But scientific associations and organizations denounce this theory saying that there is absolutely no good science to support it. Respected authors Dr. Fredrick J. Stare, M.D., and Elizabeth Whelan described this blood type diet in their book, *Fad-Free Nutrition*:

"It contains just enough scientific-sounding nonsense, carefully woven into a complex theory, to actually seem convincing to the uninitiated. . . . Browsing through what at first glance appears to be a fairly impressive list of references, we found none that seem to support a connection between diet and blood type. . . . Selecting the blood type gene as the same one that governs food and digestive capabilities is a purely arbitrary and we think irresponsible decision. He could just as easily have chosen to link food with eye color—and he would have been no farther off target . . . This outrageous theory is nothing short of sheer nonsense."

Getting the picture? Truly, a revolution is in order!

Here's a little insight into why all that meat and dairy messes with our systems. In a fascinating book called *The Pleasure Trap*, authors Douglas J. Lisle, Ph.D., and Alan Goldhamer, D.C., explain that "the solution to the modern mystery of weight management is surprisingly simple: Our modern diet is artificially concentrated, and this artificial concentration causes our calorie counting machinery to make errors." They explain that our ancestors consumed no more than 20 percent fat, since most of what they ate was vegetables and fruits, nuts and seeds, and occasionally wild game (which had only about 15 percent fat).

> But in the modern environment, our diets are replete with artificially high fat foods, whose fat percentages are typically between 35 and 80 percent! Butter, eggs, ice cream, burgers, fried foods, and other high fat animal and processed foods have fat percentages far above those of a natural diet. The modern fast food cheeseburger derived from hormone-implanted cattle living in feedlots is typically 60 to 70 percent fat—many times more fat than its wild game counterpart. Because fat is calorically concentrated, a high fat diet has an unnatural degree of caloric density. This unnatural concentration causes mistakes by our innate calorie counting machinery.

We have within us "nutrient receptors"—our natural calorie-counting mechanism—that tell our brains when we are satiated, and therefore when to stop eating. Note that animals in the wild never overeat. This is because they are eating their natural diet and so their internal calorie counting/satiation mechanisms are in place. But nature never figured on massive advertising campaigns glorifying fast food and steak dinners, and so when we answer the persistent calls of those ads, our nature-born internal receptors get thrown off. When we consume an unnaturally high amount of concentrated calories, our brain misreads the caloric value, which leads to overeating. It's like our internal check and balance system is thrown out of whack by a diet that nature never intended.

The authors also explain that the human body is designed to consume plant-based food, which is rich in fiber and has all the nutrients we need. The fiber inherent in whole grains, beans, fruits, and vegetables signals the "stretch receptors" in our belly to tell us that we are full. The stretch receptors work in tandem with the nutrient receptors to guide our instincts in getting the perfect number of calories. We need not worry about consciously counting calories, because if we are eating our nature-intended plant-based diet, the body does it for us.

> We need not worry about consciously counting calories, because if we are eating our nature-intended plant-based diet, the body does it for us.

Meat and dairy products—even if natural and free range—are inherently concentrated foods and beyond the bounds of what we should be eating. Those foods are so appealing because they give us the greatest amount of pleasure (a signal in the brain) and provide the greatest dietary reward (meaning the most amount of calories concentrated in one place) with the least amount of effort (which is good if you are a caveman scrounging for food).

In nature, this ensured that we would, say, pick ripe fruit over unripe, choose bananas for calories over celery. But the manipulation of food (by the food industry, which wants you to get hooked on its products) to increase richness beyond what is natural has caused our pleasure circuits to be hijacked, or tricked, by artificial stimulation.

And I have to share with you this mind-blowing tidbit about chicken, because so many people think chicken is a lean meat and good for weight watching. According to the nonprofit group Farm Forward, changes in gene selection for fast weight gain (along with no exercise and a constant supply of high-energy food) has increased the fat content and decreased the protein of chicken meat. They cite a study of UK chicken meat by scientists at the Institute of Brain Chemistry and Human Nutrition in London. That study reports that even though people tend to think of chicken as a protein-rich food, today's chickens are likely to have more fat than protein! In some cases, the chickens we eat may even be technically obese. As one of the researchers, Dr. Yiqun Wang, stated in the journal *Public Health Nutrition*, "This situation raises concerns for animal welfare as well as for human nutrition: does eating obesity cause obesity in the consumer?" Eating obese chickens can cause obese humans? Ach. Skip the chicken, please.

There's more. When you consume a lot of meat, your body produces an excess of uric acid. Uric acid is a waste product in the liver's metabolism of DNA, and when you eat too much meat, your body isn't able to eliminate it. This can cause gout, an extremely painful inflammation of the joints. The buildup of uric acid can also cause kidney stones, another painful occurrence you can prevent by eating a lot of fiber and avoiding meat and dairy. When you eat a lot of animal protein, your urine's pH balance becomes acidic, which makes uric acid less soluble and more likely to crystallize and form stones in your kidneys.

And finally, a high-animal-protein, low-carb diet leads to constipation and poor intestinal health. You need fiber to bulk up your intestinal contents so the rings of muscle in your gut wall have something to push against to move things along. Not only is fiber vital in the formation of stools, but it also speeds up the amount of time it takes to eliminate the waste. You don't want all that waste hanging out in your body, and not just because of the bloat and extra pounds it puts on. By not eliminating regularly, you increase your risk for colon cancer, appendicitis, diverticulosis, and hemorrhoids.

Extra Lean: Use smaller dishes so that you aren't filling up a huge plate with oversize portions. I like using a small pasta bowl as my main dish.

Remember, neither meat nor dairy nor eggs nor fish has any fiber. And without fiber, our bodies simply don't work correctly. Not only do we get constipated or experience diarrhea, but we also get fat. Today's prevailing diet of burgers, cheesy pizzas, chicken wings, and the like packs too many calories into too small a space for us to feel full at the right time, say Lisle and Goldhamer; it throws off the complex set of neural circuits that is the mechanism of satiety.

But there is an answer: we don't have to rely on willpower or white knuckle restraint as long we consume the appropriate foods—a varied, whole foods, plant-based diet.

Removing the culprit of high-density fat found in animal protein is key. (It's important to note here that even so-called lean meats are at least 20 percent fat and cause trouble to the body.) The authors assure us that in this way, the body will "naturally shed excessive fat and restore the body to health and fitness."

Extra Lean: Have some vinegar (about 2 teaspoons) with your meals; it's calorie free and good for you. It blocks the spike in blood sugar after a meal, and slows down the speed at which food leaves the stomach, keeping you feeling full longer.

Dr. Neal Barnard, founder of the Physicians Committee for Responsible Medicine, in his book *Breaking the Food Seduction*, further explains how animal protein gets a hold of our cravings in this way:

An attraction to any fatty food makes some biological sense. Fat happens to be the most calorie-dense part of any food we eat. . . . Presumably, as our species evolved, those people who knew a calorie when they saw one—that is, those who were attracted to fattier foods—would be more likely to survive in times of scarcity. If that taste for fat leads us to the occasional nut, seed, or olive, no harm is done. But nature never figured that this same attraction would lead us to prefer hamburgers, fried chicken, and other dangerously fatty foods.

Scientists believe that, once we get used to fatty foods as a result of their being on our plate day after day, we come to prefer them and tend to seek them out. . . . Tests suggest that meat may have subtle drug-like qualities. . . . What appears to be happening is that, as meat touches your tongue, opiates are released in the brain, rewarding you—rightly or wrongly—for your calorie-dense food choice and propelling you toward making it a habit. . . . The good news is that once a meat habit has been decidedly broken for a few weeks it fades from memory surprisingly easily.

Barnard adds that, curiously, meat stimulates insulin release. Whereas it is common knowledge that simple carbohydrates cause the body to release a lot of insulin, thereby setting off a rise in blood sugar, recent studies show that meat also causes a "distinct, sometimes surprising, insulin spike. In fact, beef and cheese cause a bigger insulin release than pasta, and fish produces a bigger insulin release than popcorn."

> **Recent studies show that meat also causes a "distinct, sometimes surprising, insulin spike. In fact, beef and cheese cause a bigger insulin release than pasta."**

But, yeah, what *about* fish? I hear you asking; isn't that a good choice for weight loss? Let's bust that myth right now: no, fish is not the best option for weight loss. Fish still has fat in it, and 15 to 30 percent of that fat is saturated fat, and that's not good. True, it's better than beef or chicken (50 percent and 20–30 percent respectively), but why go there when you're much better off all around with plant foods? Calorically, fat is fat. There are 9 calories per fat gram, no matter where the fat comes from, as opposed to 4 calories per gram of carbohydrate. And if you don't think that fish fat piles up on the bod, take a look at the well-padded tummies and thighs of folks who live in the Arctic and live primarily on salmon. They are not skinny folk. And sadly, there is just about no place in our oceans that is unaffected by industrial pollution. So much seafood offered these days is contaminated with mercury, pesticides, and PCBs— toxic chemicals that were used in electrical equipment, paints, and hydraulic fluid before they were banned as carcinogenic pollutants.

If you know where to look and who to trust, it is not that difficult to separate the scientific wheat from the chaff. One of the few physicians to help people take weight off and keep it off in peer-reviewed scientific studies is Dr. Dean Ornish, who notes that although fad diets work for a little while, according to a government study, "two-thirds of people gained back all the weight they lost within a year, and 97 percent gained it all back within five years. The secret to losing weight and keeping it off is a diet that is delicious, life affirming, and sustainable: vegetarian. And better still is vegan."

So today, you will start eating two out of your three meals without animals, and nudge yourself even farther along the path. You'll be getting loads of fiber, which amps your metabolism, a lot less fat and saturated fat, and none of the health problems that go along with eating animal foods.

Just so you know how very safe and established this diet is, note that the American Dietetic Association has looked at all the studies that have been done and concluded not just that a vegetarian diet is as healthy as one that includes meat, but that "[v]egetarians have been reported to have lower body mass indices than nonvegetarians, as well as lower rates of death from ischemic heart disease; vegetarians also show lower blood cholesterol levels; lower blood pressure; and lower rates of hypertension, type 2 diabetes, and prostate and colon cancer." That's right—it's not just that vegetarians tend to be slimmer, but they also suffer from lower rates of most of the biggest chronic diseases that plague us.

Deborah, a reader who wrote to me, says this:

When I started my journey toward moving away from meat and dairy I weighed 168 pounds. I've already lost 38 pounds, and it was easy. (And the arthritis in my knees is gone.) It is amazing how when you eat good foods you crave good foods! I used to be addicted to chicken Parmesan and I replaced it with eggplant Parm with nondairy cheese! I eat brown rice and salad with raw vegetables every day for lunch instead of chicken sandwiches and french fries. I love the Morningstar Farms [vegan] chick'n strips and Morningstar veggie burgers [available at most good supermarkets nationwide]. I am still trying new things every single day. I recently tried Gardein [plant-based] meats as well as Daiya animal-free cheese. I cannot believe how wonderful these products are! I make my own version of mac and cheese with Daiya cheese and almond milk and no one knows the difference! I make it for my friends and family and they don't realize there's nothing animal in there.

There's all the *why* you'll ever need. Now go try a black bean tostada with salsa (hold the sour cream and cheese) or a hearty lentil soup, or maybe some grilled veggie sausages with a big salad on the side. Go to the recipes at the back of this book, or to a favorite meatless cookbook, and pick out a lunch that looks good to you. Enjoy its heartiness and know that your body is really going to change for the better.

So, what are you going to do today?

✓ Drink lots of water.
✓ Eat a hearty breakfast.
✓ Eat an apple.
✓ Just for today, say no to your poison.
✓ Go a little nuts.
✓ Trade up the milk and butter.
✓ Put a little flax on it.
✓ Do a deep dive for five.
✓ Switch up your drinks.
✓ Make lunch without animal products.

DAY 11.

Take Your Vites

TODAY WE'RE BACK TO ADDING SOMETHING, AND THAT SOMETHING IS very simple. Today you are going to pop a little vitamin or two so that you can move forward in your Lean, knowing you have everything you need in terms of the basics.

Did your mom ever tell you to take your vitamins? If she did, she was probably right. Obviously, your best source of nutrients is whole foods like beans and grains, fruits and vegetables, and with this Lean approach you are already eating healthy (or healthier) meals every day, but you could still miss out on some essential nutrition, at least while you are still finding your way.

Sometimes circumstances just don't allow us to eat optimally every day—you may not have time to shop thoughtfully or cook at home; or you may be in a rush and simply can't get your hands on something decent to eat. Whatever the reason, there may be gaps in your diet that preclude you from getting everything you need, and it can't hurt to have a little insurance.

Also, it's not all a matter of what we choose to eat. Our soil is so degraded from overusing it for agricultural purposes that food isn't what it used to be. The increasing toxicity in our environment has caused the nutritional quality of our food to decline. Those of you growing your own food in organic and ideal conditions may be exempt. Still, I err on the side of caution.

Aside from ensuring you get all the nutrients you need, vitamin supplements can also aid the weight loss process. This is because poor nutrition will leave you feeling fatigued and craving food, likely fattening comfort food. If your cells aren't getting what they need to nourish them, you simply won't have the energy to stay focused on your plan, making the necessary shifts in your diet while adding in sufficient exercise. Even if you ultimately decide to go without taking any vitamins (and you certainly can), you would do well to consider the following, at least while you are still finding your footing. I think you might find you quickly feel a boost of energy and a sense of wellness.

Multivitamin

A multivitamin is at the very least an inexpensive nutrition insurance policy. It covers a broad base of vital nutrients and can help to rectify most of the gaps in your diet (even though I'm hoping you will take the Lean to heart and eat super well!). If finances allow, choose a food-grown, mostly organic one, as those supplements have the nutrients compressed from actual healthful foods rather than being chemically engineered. It's best not to take a multi that has both iron and calcium in it, as the iron can block the uptake of calcium. Iron can also make you feel nauseated or upset your stomach, so you'll probably do better taking it separately if you decide you need it. If you hate taking pills, try a liquid supplement. And if you are taking a capsule or soft gel, be sure the coating isn't made from gelatin, since that comes from the skin and bones of pigs and cows or horses' hooves. (Ach, gross, I know. But I thought you'd like to know.)

B$_{12}$

The B vitamins are good for the nervous and digestive systems. They are easily lost in the refining or cooking process and can be diminished by heavy sweating, or drinking a lot of alcohol, tea, or coffee.

Vegans sometimes lack vitamin B_{12}, and there's an interesting story about why. The common story is that vegetables just don't have B_{12}, but that's not necessarily true. It's a matter of how sanitized our food supply has become. B_{12} is produced by microorganisms (such as bacteria) that no longer make their way into vegetables that are cleansed of all "dirt." Animals, on the other hand, eat and drink a lot of dirt throughout the day; the B_{12} comes from the bacteria in their digestive tract and is then passed on to the carnivores who ingest them.

As well, the National Institutes of Health advise that older adults, people with pernicious anemia, and those with reduced levels of stomach acidity or intestinal disorders may have difficulty absorbing B_{12}. The NIH also notes that the prevalence of deficiency in young adults might be greater than previously assumed. In any case, it's a good idea to supplement your diet, and it's essential for someone following a plant-based diet. The Institute of Medicine recommends taking 2.4 micrograms per day, although if you are eating a lot of fortified foods you will likely be covered. Signs of B-vitamin deficiency are memory loss, disorientation, and tingling in the arms and legs. As an interesting (and potentially very promising) aside, many people who think they are suffering from dementia or Alzheimer's might actually be lacking in B_{12}, a situation that can be addressed and reversed. It's suggested that B_{12} taken under the tongue—a spray version, for example, is absorbed better.

Iron

The most healthful sources of iron are greens and all kinds of beans—green leafy veggies like kale and collards (not spinach, surprisingly, because the iron in spinach is not well absorbed), and beans like navy or black beans. These foods are also abundant in calcium and other important minerals. But if blood tests show you are low in iron or are anemic, you might want to try supplementing until you hit your stride with your upgraded eating patterns. Taking extra iron is vital for some of us, especially women of childbearing age who may be anemic because of heavy periods. We need iron to make hemoglobin, which carries life-giving oxygen to the cells. Iron is involved in the production of energy from the metabolism of food. Some of the symptoms of anemia are fatigue, gas, constipation, cold intolerance, and decreased resistance to infection. If you are low on iron, your ability to work and exercise is likely compromised.

That said, you don't want to have too much iron in your body, because excess iron can help produce free radicals (which, again, cause all sorts of problems like aging, heart disease, and cancer). Next time you are at the doctor, have him or her take a look at your hemoglobin count; it is best at the low end of normal.

Vitamin D

You've likely heard a lot of noise about vitamin D lately, and it's all good news. Vitamin D is a nutrient that we get from food, and it's a hormone that our bodies make. It's not found abundantly in any particular food, so it's a good idea to supplement it. Research over the past decade has shown that vitamin D plays a much bigger role in fighting disease than previously thought; it boosts your immune system in a big way and reduces the risk of many serious illnesses. It's best obtained from 15 minutes a day of exposure to natural sunlight, but if sunshine isn't abundantly available or you want to take care to prevent skin damage, take a supplement.

Research over the past decade has shown that vitamin D plays a much bigger role in fighting disease than previously thought.

The Harvard School of Public Health recommends taking 1000IU to 2000IU per day, while recent clinical research shows that the higher dose is more appropriate to optimum health. Vitamin D is essential for calcium absorption and for bone mineralization, but an even more exciting property is that vitamin D is helpful in preventing many degenerative diseases, including heart disease, some kinds of cancer (the evidence is strongest for colon cancer), some autoimmune diseases, multiple sclerosis, infectious diseases, and even nuisance illnesses like flu and the common cold.

Omega-3

You've undoubtedly heard about the benefits of omega-3 fatty acids; they are essential for controlling blood clotting and building cell membranes in the brain, and they are associated with lowering the risk of heart disease and stroke. Many people take fish oil, and so I asked Dr. Neal Barnard what his take on it is. This is what he says:

> Vegetable sources are fine and are preferable to fish oils. There are only two essential fats, and both come from plant sources.
>
> 1. ALA (alpha-linolenic acid) is a basic omega-3 fat. In the body, it can be converted to the other omega-3s the body needs. So, in the human body, ALA (which is a chain of 18 carbons) is lengthened to EPA (20 carbons) and DHA (22 carbons). ALA occurs in small amounts in beans, vegetables, and fruits, and this is probably all the body needs. If people want more, they will find it in walnuts, soy products, and, in high concentration, in flaxseeds and flax oil.
>
>   The problem seems to arise when people eat lots of other fats that compete with ALA. That is, fats found in many junk foods such as cottonseed oil compete with ALA for the enzymes that would normally convert ALA to the various other omega-3 fats. These competitors slow down ALA's conversion to other fats. This is the reason some people push fish oil; it has a variety of preformed omega-3 fats that the fish produced from ALA. Our bodies will do the same, if we let it happen.
>
>   Recently, vegan sources of longer-chain omega-3s have come on the market. They contain EPA and DHA.

There is no advantage to fish oil over these products. But none of them are necessary, so far as I can see.

2. The other essential fat is called linoleic acid, and it is widely available throughout the plant kingdom, so finding it is not a problem.

Fish fats do contain omega-3. But 70 percent or more of the fat in fish is *not* omega-3. Rather, it is a mixture of saturated and unsaturated fats that do the body no good at all. This is why fish does not reduce cholesterol for most people.

So, in summary, Dr. Barnard says that if you are eating a well-rounded diet including flax, soy, and walnuts, you probably don't need anything in addition. But if you feel like you'd like some extra protection, you can get an omega-3 supplement made of algae, which is where the fish get their omegas (nothing like cutting out the middle man!).

Probiotics

Probiotics are often referred to as "friendly bacteria"; they are microorganisms that help with digestion and nutrient absorption, and they protect your body against "bad bacteria" that can find its way into your gut. Whenever we take antibiotics, the "good bacteria" are wiped out along with the bad, leaving us without the helpful army of beneficial microflora to fight off illnesses and balance our intestinal environment. Remember, if you eat meat, chicken, dairy, and/or eggs, the animals were often fed antibiotics, so even if you haven't been on a course of antibiotics yourself, you are probably ingesting some.

You might find it interesting, or should I say frightening, that over 70 percent of antibiotics produced in this country go to livestock to make them grow faster and stay alive long enough (the crowded conditions in factory farms make them sick) to be profitably fattened for slaughter.

Taking probiotics replenishes the good guys and fights off

unfriendly pathogens. They may also be helpful to people who suffer from irritable bowel syndrome, Crohn's disease, and urinary infections.

In terms of weight management, you might be surprised to see how your stomach flattens out once you have your gut bacteria back to a healthy place and the bloat goes away. Choose a probiotic with as high a count of live bacteria as you can find. Remember, too, to keep your probiotics in the fridge, as they are living organisms.

EATING FOR A HEALTHY GUT

Dr. Michael Greger also tells us this:

There is a way to boost the good bacteria in the colon without probiotics: by feeding them the right food. Fiber. Our friendly flora digestion of fiber yields a short-chain fatty acid called *butyrate*. Butyrate seems to have a broad anti-inflammatory effect on our system. And we can produce more on our own by eating more plant foods. (Many studies have shown that vegetarians harbor more good bacteria than anyone else, and vegetarian fecal samples show the highest number of copies of butyrate-producing genes.)

Other than fiber, what else do plants make that animals don't that could help account for how dramatically slimmer those who eat plant-based diets tend to be? Phytonutrients. Mammals, including humans, harbor two main phyla of friendly gut bacteria: Bacteroidetes and the Firmicutes. In terms of obesity, though, one appears friendlier than the other. There is mounting evidence that gut flora in healthy people is different from the flora in obese people: Firmicutes significantly outnumber Bacteroidetes in those who are overweight or obese. Here's a little mnemonic device for keeping them straight: fatter Firmicutes and bonier Bacteroidetes. Obese individuals appear to have more Firmicutes than Bacteroidetes in their guts.

If you put people on a diet for a year you can actually change the proportion. Certain antibiotics may trigger obesity by mucking around down there. How can we improve the ratio? Well, a class of phytonutrients called polyphenols do two things: they are the preferred food of Bacteroidetes while at the same time suppressing the growth of Firmicutes. Maybe that's why the use of vinegar has been recommended for thousands of years for weight loss. What's it often made out of? Grapes (red wine vinegar) or apples (apple cider vinegar). Both grapes and apples are packed with polyphenols. The weight-lowering property of fruits, green tea, and wine vinegar in obese people may be partly related to their polyphenol content, which changes the gut flora.

Naysayers who disbelieve the power of phytonutrients often point to studies showing that up to 85 percent of those wonderful blue anthocyanins in blueberries end up in your colon unabsorbed. But that may be where some of the magic happens.

So basically, yes, our gut flora help determine our weight, but the answer is not necessarily to take probiotics but to feed the bacteria we have the right stuff (I do recommend probiotics after courses of oral antibiotics, but that's a special case).

It's a good thing you are drinking your 8 glasses of water, too, because water acts as a solvent for many vitamins and minerals, and is also in charge of carrying nutrients into and wastes out of cells so the body operates properly. Here's how I'd suggest you handle your supplements.

Take your multi, vitamin D, and omega-3 with breakfast or lunch. The fat in your food will help carry the fat-soluble vitamins to your cells, so don't just take these on an empty stomach or with just water. Take your probiotics on an empty stomach (the acid produced during meal digestion is there in part to kill off harmful bacteria and so can be counterproductive if you are trying to sneak some good bacteria past your defenses). Take iron at least two hours away from your multi and before a meal. You can take the B_{12} anytime you'd like. Out of all these, a multi and the D are the essentials that will go far in protecting you, and from what I've learned from the leading nutritional scientists, they are well worth the investment. The multi likely has enough B_{12} in it, so unless you think you are running particularly low, just take that.

Taking your vitamins is an easy step and an important one, but it's not nearly as important for your health as eating well! There is no beating a diverse diet of beans, whole grains, tubers, veggies, fruits, nuts, and seeds and steering clear of sugar and super-processed foods.

So, what are you going to do today?

- ✓ Drink lots of water.
- ✓ Eat a hearty breakfast.
- ✓ Eat an apple.
- ✓ Just for today, say no to your poison.
- ✓ Go a little nuts.
- ✓ Trade up the milk and butter.
- ✓ Put a little flax on it.
- ✓ Do a deep dive for five.
- ✓ Switch up your drinks.
- ✓ Make lunch without animal products.
- ✓ Take your vites.

DAY 12.

Add In Some Exercise

YOU MAY HAVE NOTICED THAT WE'VE BEEN FOCUSING ON FOODS, BUT they're only part of the Lean plan. Today is your day to get moving! No new foods today, just some booty shaking.

If you've been a reluctant exerciser, I want you to just take a deep breath, push yourself out the door, and do something, anything, to get your heart rate up a bit. If you already exercise, I want you to lean in a little further and up your program.

I remember that when I first wanted to start exercising, I was at a complete loss for what to do. I didn't grow up playing sports, and I was extremely sluggish. When I started eating better, my energy level changed, and I knew it was time to start expending some of that energy. So I just walked out my front door and strolled around the block. It felt good to be outside, breathing the fresh air and checking out the neighborhood.

I did that for a week, and then extended my walk to about a mile, all the while upping my speed. Sometimes I walked with a friend, sometimes I listened to music or lectures (back then I had a Sony Walkman and cassettes!), and I always brought my dog along. I kept doing that until I got bored (a few months had gone by), and then a couple of times a week, I would drive to a local hiking area.

Extra Lean: Get a buddy to work out with; it'll make the sessions more fun and harder to cancel. And by the way, an interesting recent study showed that if your friends are slim, you are more likely to be slim. So bring your friends along on your program to lose weight and get healthy, so you can all inspire and influence each other!

By that time, I viewed myself as more of an outdoorsy person (amazing how quickly perceptions of ourselves can change!) and I welcomed being out in the hills with nature. My hikes were slow going at first, but before I knew it, I was speeding up the hill with determination on my face and a ridiculously happy dog at my side.

My friend Lisa started out running and then started training for half marathons. Pretty soon she had moved on to triathlons. As she put it, "I experienced a high like I had never felt before, and the weight just started coming off. I built more muscle and got stronger and completely reshaped my body."

Of course, you don't have to go there. My point is simply that movement begets movement. When you nudge yourself to move even just a little, you get used to the exertion pretty quickly. And then exercise becomes a natural and steady part of your daily routine.

A lovely woman named Tammy wrote to me with this to say about the motivation to keep active:

> *I guess if I could give a tip or secret on how to lean in, it's just to keep leaning in! People seem to fly from one extreme to the next, but it's really difficult to live life that way. Seeing the success as you lean in gives you more incentive to keep leaning in! It works! And I'm enjoying every second of it!*

Let's take a look at how exercise changes your body.
Exercise and weight loss are two components of a seemingly

very simple equation: exercise assists weight loss and management because physical activity increases calorie burn, and the calorie deficits this creates, over time, cause weight loss. That's the straightforward explanation, but exercise is really much more than mere calorie burn. Its proven health benefits are numerous: increased metabolism, extra energy, even the prevention of cognitive decline: a recent study by the Harvard Medical School shows that just 30 minutes of moderately vigorous daily exercise will extend your mental clarity by as much as seven years as you get older.

It's also a proven way to combat mild to moderate depression and anxiety, which also affect your weight.

Aerobic exercise (sometimes referred to as cardio exercise) is the kind that doctors and researchers are constantly reminding people to do on a daily basis. Aerobic exercise encompasses a variety of different physical activities, but in a nutshell it's really just the name for any kind of physical activity that causes your heart and lungs to work more than they do when you're resting. Aerobic activity boosts the amount of oxygen in your blood, elevates your heart rate, expands the capillaries in your body, and stimulates the release of endorphins. These complex interactions activate all kinds of health advantages in your body, but they're also responsible for one very simple effect: weight loss, especially when combined with balanced eating.

Extra Lean: Listen to some rockin' tunes if you are working out in the gym; the music will distract you from feeling tired or bored, and a recent study showed that men who work out to music go 11 percent longer than without.

How Much?

Busy lives leave many people feeling that they have very little time to work in physical activity. But only a half hour per day is all it takes to enhance weight loss, and for that small time investment you get a lifelong rate of return.

I can hear some of you resisting. You don't have a half hour a day, you say? I assure you, you do. You must. Even if you are taking care of small children or working long hours at your job, you *can* find a half hour for exercise. Instead of staying at your desk through lunch, get out for a short walk. (Then eat, of course; I don't want you to miss a meal!) At night, instead of plunking yourself down in front of the television, do a little jog to your favorite show. Or jump rope during the commercials! (See below.) Instead of getting lost on Facebook or checking e-mail, pop in an exercise DVD or turn on the Wii and get fit. If you want to find the time, you can and you will.

> **Extra Lean:** Do some stretching while you are watching the telly; reach for your toes, do some side bends and lower back twists. Throw in some push-ups and crunches. It'll keep you in a positive body-conscious state while also crowding out snack time.

Nathan wrote in to tell me that he took small steps and is really feeling the results.

> *I bought a bike and go for regular rides, nothing serious but just a relaxing trek along a bike path in the city. I walk to work, it's only a block, but on my way home I will walk in a 10-block loop. Just to make sure I'm more active than I was last week, or last month or last year.*

Exercise is a paradox: the boost of mental energy you get from it more than compensates for the actual time you spend doing it by increasing your mental clarity, which in turn boosts your overall productivity, allowing you to do more in less time.

Experts at organizations like the Centers for Disease Control and Prevention (CDC) and the American College of Sports Medicine (ACSM) advise that 150 minutes per week is an adequate amount of exercise for moderate weight loss and maintenance. You can divide up the 150 minutes into several different time segments according to your schedule. To get to 150 minutes per week, you could do:

- 1¼ hours (75 minutes) of vigorous aerobic activity twice a week . . . OR
- 50 minutes both moderate and intense activities 3 times a week . . . OR
- 3 daily 10-minute intervals of moderate to intense activity spaced throughout your day . . . OR
- 25 minutes of moderate activity 6 days per week (this is my favorite equation, as it's steady and fits into a daily routine well)

The numbers of possible combinations to choose from make exercise doable on practically anyone's schedule. The only caveat? The CDC and ACSM emphasize that the activity should be spaced out throughout the week for best results, if possible, and that each interval should last for at least 10 minutes.

> **Extra Lean:** Purchase a pedometer; seeing how many steps you are taking, and challenging yourself to reach at least 10,000 per day, will keep you motivated and moving.

What kind of results can you expect to see from 150 minutes per week of exercise? The Duke University STRRIDE experiment found remarkable differences over the course of the eight-month study they conducted on participants who exercised versus those who didn't. Participants who did 30 minutes of brisk walking daily lost 2 percent of their body fat and gained .7 percent lean muscle. However, all the sedentary study participants who were restricted from exercising *gained* weight, resulting in bigger waistlines (by .8 percent) and increased body fat (.5 percent).

As you'd expect, participants who increased the intensity and duration of weekly exercise got the best results of all in the form of increased fat loss and muscle gain. These participants lost more than double the amount (4.9 percent) of their body fat and gained twice the amount of lean muscle mass (1.4 percent) in comparison.

> **Extra Lean:** Celebrate when you feel like you've lost a little weight: get a mani-pedi, or buy yourself a little something special (not food, though).

What's Moderate, What's Vigorous

Exercise intensity is classified broadly as moderate or vigorous, and unless you buy and use a personal heart rate monitor, these terms are a bit subjective. The Mayo Clinic offers these handy tips for determining how your body's responses are correlated with the intensity of the physical activity that you're doing.

Light exercise intensity feels undemanding, with no noticeable changes in breathing.

- You don't break a sweat (unless it's very hot or humid).
- You can easily carry on a full conversation or even sing.

Moderate exercise intensity feels somewhat hard; you can tell that you're working.

- Your breathing quickens, but you're not out of breath.
- You develop a light sweat after about 10 minutes of activity.
- You can carry on a conversation, but you can't sing.

Vigorous exercise intensity feels challenging; now you *know* you're working.

- Your breathing is deep and rapid.
- You develop a sweat after a few minutes of activity.
- You can't say more than a few words without pausing for breath.

Thanks, Mayo Clinic, for that great info on fitness intensity!

Any physical activity that you can think of is aerobic, and a list of what "counts" would be endless. It doesn't even have to be a traditional sporting or exercise activity; even vigorous household chores count if you don't have time to go for a run or hop on a bike. The National Heart, Lung, and Blood Institute offers this guide to choosing specific activities that'll get your heart rate up.

Moderate Level Activities

Washing/waxing your car for 45–60 minutes
Washing windows or floors for 45–60 minutes
Gardening for 30–45 minutes
Pushing a stroller 1.5 miles in 30 minutes or less
Walking 2 miles in 30 minutes, or 15 minutes per mile
Stairwalking for 15 minutes
Volleyball for 45–60 minutes
Walking 1.75 miles in 35 minutes, or 20 minutes per mile
Basketball for 30 minutes
Biking for 5 miles in 30 minutes
Jumping rope for 15 minutes
Running 1.5 miles in 15 minutes, a 10-minute mile

Vigorous Level Activities (requires only 25 minutes or less, according to the CDC)

Racewalking, jogging, or running 5 mph or faster
Roller or inline skating

Biking uphill
Karate or other martial arts
Bicycling 10 mph or faster
Jumping rope (intense rate)
Heavy gardening (continuous digging or hoeing)
Hiking uphill with a backpack [or, if you're more than
    50 pounds over the ideal weight for your height, without
    the backpack!]
Jumping jacks
Singles tennis
Walking quickly up a hill

Extra Lean: Adopt a pet (assuming you have time to spend with him or her). People who have dogs tend to be more active and less obese than those who don't. You'll also feel less anxious if you have a dog or cat, and that means less of the stress hormone cortisol. Since cortisol seems to direct fat to the belly, it's a good thing to cozy up with your critter to chill, or better yet, shake off the angst on a vigorous walk!

Calorie Expenditure

Some basic information to keep in mind:

- Increasing calories burned is the most basic way that exercise stimulates weight loss, but there's a lot of room for variation in how many calories you burn doing any specific activity.
- The amount of calories burned depends more on how much the activity elevates your heart rate compared with its resting rate, not the type of activity; however, some ex-

ercises naturally require more movement or are more
intense than others.

- Calorie expenditure also depends on several other factors,
  like gender, age, current weight, intensity, and duration of
  activity.
- The lower your weight, the fewer calories you burn, so as
  you gradually lose weight, you should increase your level
  of activity accordingly to continue to reap benefits.

Exercise is far more effective at helping you lose weight when
it's combined with consistent dietary changes. Since 1994, the National Weight Control Registry has studied the weight loss strategies
of more than 5,000 people who have lost more than 30 pounds and
sustained the loss long term: well over 90 percent of all successful
participants combined diet with exercise, and walking was the most
commonly reported exercise.

Remember that it's possible to overeat and wipe out the weight
loss benefits of any exercise you've done. It takes 30 minutes of walking to burn just over 100 calories; it takes only 30 seconds or less to
eat 300 calories.

Getting Started

The key to exercise is consistency, and experts agree that people who
exercise in the morning seem to be better able to stick with their program. Scheduling your exercise in the morning allows you to do it
before all the pressures of work or family begin to build up. But if
you can't exercise in the morning, don't worry: while morning exercise is best for consistency, evidence suggests that early evening exercise, around 6 P.M., is best for overall performance.

Walking is the easiest exercise to take up. It costs nothing except a decent pair of walking shoes, and you can do it anywhere. If
you're at a beginner fitness level, start with a brisk 10-minute walk
every day, in the morning before breakfast, on your lunch break, or

after dinner. Choose a destination: whether it's a natural landmark like a lake or a hill, or a city park, having a clear end point in mind is a big help. From there, you can build up stamina gradually; walking up a hill or on a rougher trail adds a challenge.

Bicycling and jumping rope are also good beginner-to-intermediate exercises. You can get weighted jump ropes at any fitness store or online to increase the upper body workout and make it a more challenging session, and you may already have a bike. Consistently increase the intensity: if you jump rope for 10 minutes this week, do it for 15 the next. If you ride your bike 2 miles, next week ride it 4. You'll be surprised at how quickly an activity that used to feel difficult becomes easy, and that's when it's time to up things a notch.

If you get bored with the activity you're doing, switch it up! It's normal to want novelty in your exercise routine. Many people misinterpret feeling bored with an activity as a sign that they just don't like to exercise when nothing could be further than the truth. Boredom is just an indication that it's time to try a new activity, or to add a new layer of challenge to the one you're already doing. This is also true of choosing which form of exercise to start your program with: if walking is unappealing, play tennis, or ask a friend to walk with you. If bicycling is unattractive, take a martial arts class instead.

The ideas that are most important to take away are these: exercise is accessible to anyone regardless of current fitness level, schedule, or cost. It's really just a matter of starting in the way that's best for you. The biggest barrier to starting and sustaining a exercise program is the mental one. Do it daily; establishing a new habit takes time, but the health and weight loss results are well worth it. Start with something easy today, but just move. If you are already moving, challenge yourself a little more. This program is all about pushing yourself a little farther along, making the tweaks that will continue to help you lose weight—*and* aid your sense of accomplishment and growth!

So, what are you going to do today?

✓ Drink lots of water.
✓ Eat a hearty breakfast.
✓ Eat an apple.
✓ Just for today, say no to your poison.
✓ Go a little nuts.
✓ Trade up the milk and butter.
✓ Put a little flax on it.
✓ Do a deep dive for five.
✓ Switch up your drinks.
✓ Make lunch without animal products.
✓ Take your vites.
✓ Add in some exercise.

DAY 13.

Change Up Your Cheese

BACK ON DAY 6 WE TALKED ABOUT MILKS AND BUTTERS THAT AREN'T animal derived. Today we're going to find great alternatives to that other source of true dairy pleasure: cheese.

I can hear you grumbling. You think this little tweak may not be so fun. I'm guessing that if you are like a great majority of Americans you love cheese just about more than anything in life, and you think you could never give it up. You don't *want* to give it up. And even if you wanted to give it up, you couldn't, because when you get the hankering, you are truly possessed by some crazy urge for that ooey, gooey, creamy texture and you simply cannot say no.

Perhaps it's even your favorite addiction. I get it, and I used to feel the same way. Here's the good news: you don't have to give up cheese!

(Are you doing the dance of joy? Dance away, because this is all part of the crowding out plan.)

Here's what we're going to do: instead of cheese made from cow or goat's milk, we are simply going to slide you over to nondairy cheese. You will still get the great creamy texture you love, the added richness to your favorite foods, but without all the problems that go along with eating dairy.

And by the way, can we talk about what it really means to eat cheese? You are consuming the breast milk of a 1,500-pound animal! I mean, imagine a friend of yours inviting you to her house for pizza by saying, "Come on over for dinner; I used my breast milk to make some cheese for the pizza, and I think you will really like the taste of it!"

Um, no thank you.

It's easy enough to see why that's not such a great idea, because obviously, our breast milk is only meant for our babies for a short time in their little lives while they are rapidly growing and forming their bodies. And the breast milk of a cow, rather than a human, is okay for why exactly? Yuck.

And besides, you'll recall our earlier discussion about the fact that milk is designed to help a teeny little calf grow 1,000-plus pounds in a very short amount of time. We do not want to grow that much, thank you very much!

Okay, onward.

When you want to lose weight, dairy products (even "fat-free," "part skim," or "low-fat" versions) are your worst enemy. Let's get to the science of why we are going to make the switch from animal-based cheese to nondairy cheese. And no sacrifice, I promise.

Something to ponder: cheese consumption in America has increased hugely over the past several decades, and obesity has soared right alongside. This is no coincidence. In his breakthrough work on nutrition, T. Colin Campbell has found a clear and strong correlation between consumption of animal protein and higher body weight. A century ago, Americans consumed about 4 pounds of cheese per person per year; this amount has increased by a whopping 725 percent, to 33 pounds per person per year. That's a lot of fat and calories, which add to extra body weight.

By eating cheese, you are fighting an uphill battle to lose weight. The dairy industry, however, continues to muddy the nutritional waters by funding studies and devising clever marketing campaigns in an attempt to convince us that cheese is actually helpful for weight loss and management, and new misinformation is spread daily. Even the government is in on the act. A November 2010 *New York Times* article about Dairy Management, a marketing division of the USDA whose mission is promoting dairy products to the public in order to financially benefit farmers—mostly corporately owned factory farms, by the way (whose crops are already largely government subsidized)—reveals the ugly truth behind the misinformation campaign. Promoting increased cheese consumption has been a successful PR strategy—even if the dairy industry itself is aware that dairy isn't part of a successful weight loss plan. The *Times* article says:

> Dairy Management spent millions of dollars on research to support a national advertising campaign promoting the notion that people could lose weight by consuming more dairy products, records and interviews show. The campaign went on for four years, ending in 2007, even though other researchers—one paid by Dairy Management itself—*found no such weight-loss benefits*. (emphasis added)

So what's a weight-conscious cheese lover to do? To begin with, it's a common misconception that a plant-based diet means that you never eat cheese again—it just means you eat cheese derived from healthier sources. In any well-stocked grocery store, and increasingly many local ones, there are quite a lot of varieties of nondairy cheese, and if you've ever thought them unpalatable, it's time to reconsider.

Cheese alternatives have come a long way in terms of taste and quality, even in just the past few years, and as a result their use is becoming more widespread.

Plant-based cheeses (made from nuts, tapioca, soy, rice, or nutritional yeast) are delicious, and convey benefits that traditional dairy cheese just can't match. These healthful alternatives are generally lower in calories (though you should always read labels, as this varies according to the product), and lower in fat, especially saturated fat. Additionally, the plant-based origins of cheese alternatives means that they typically contain some fiber, which will help you feel fuller and more satiated.

Even if the nondairy cheeses don't taste absolutely delish to you upon first sampling (and they probably will!), keep giving them a chance. It takes around 21 days to change your palate, and I think you'll see that after a very short time, you'll hugely enjoy the gooey rich taste and texture of the dairyless versions of cheese. You might even find that there are so many yummy meals to be had without cheese—dairy or nondairy—that you'll just move away from it altogether. Keep leaning!

Here's what my friend Natala had to say about giving up animal-based cheeses:

> *Cheese and I had a very special relationship. I was known for throwing wine and cheese parties; I loved all kinds of cheese and could not imagine life without it. Even after finding out all of the dangers of cheese and how it was impacting my health, I still craved it. I'd soon learn that if I could just go without it completely for one month, my cravings would get less and less, and in a couple of months the lure of cheese just wasn't there anymore. I didn't really replace it, I just took it out of my diet, and filled my diet with more whole foods like greens, fruits, grains, beans. My tastes simply started to change as I let them.*

In case you didn't read Natala's full story in my last book, she not only lost over 200 pounds, but because of her change in diet, she no longer needs insulin or blood pressure and cholesterol lowering drugs—nine different drugs in all!

The Power of the Nutritional Package

With all the talk of low-fat this and low-fat that, it's important not to lose sight of some important nutritional realities. Some fat in the diet is necessary; it helps maximize the absorption of fat-soluble vitamins and phytonutrients. Remember: it's not what you eat, but what you absorb. And some fats are essential in the diet (the omega-3s and omega-6s) since our bodies can't make them. But our bodies have no need for dietary saturated fats like those found in animals, such as lard, tallow, and butterfat (from which animal cheeses are derived), and they can be downright detrimental. In fact, animal fats are both nonessential and can be damaging to your body.

You've heard the term "saturated fat" before, but what does it actually mean? In the simplest technical terms, saturated fats are fat molecules whose chemical chains are fully *saturated* with hydrogen. But the important thing to remember is that they're both completely unnecessary and harmful because they can raise the level of bad cholesterol in our blood, the number one risk factor for our number one killer, heart disease.

Extra Lean: You may have heard that sheep and goat cheeses are lower in fat or somehow closer to the composition of human milk (in the case of goat), but all the above facts remain true: all animal-derived cheeses are trouble for your waistline and can jeopardize your health.

And here's something from Dr. Michael Greger of Nutrition Facts.org:

For the waistline, soy is the best. Swapping in soy protein (in soy cheese) for cow's milk protein (in cow cheese) in people's diets has been found to cause a significant slimming in waist circumference—even if the amount of calories remains constant. People fed the cow milk protein casein saw their abdomen increase 20 to 40 square centimeters, whereas with these same diets (same number of calories) but soy protein instead of cow, one's tummy instead shrinks 10 to 15 square centimeters. Any nondairy cheese would also avoid the growth hormone problem of milk, which increases levels of a growth factor called IGF-1 in the body which facilitates the formation of new fat cells and has been particularly associated with childhood obesity.

Cheese is a very high fat food, and the fat is highly saturated. Plant-based cheese sources (nuts, soy, tapioca), on the other hand, contain little to no saturated fat, and their fiber content is an added bonus. Cheese alternatives also contain fat, but the major difference is that the fat in cheese alternatives is primarily the kind that's better for you; the mono- and polyunsaturated kinds. These fats are not associated with obesity and heart disease the way saturated fats are.

Here you'll find the nutritional profiles of a few of the most commonly available cheese alternatives. The superiority of the plant-based cheeses in terms of their overall calorie, fat, saturated fat, and cholesterol content is clear when compared directly with their dairy counterparts. Look for them in the health and natural foods aisles of your local supermarket or natural foods store.

1 ounce serving of Daiya Cheddar Style Shreds
   90 calories
   6 grams of fat, 2 of them saturated
   0 milligrams of cholesterol
   1 gram of fiber

1 ounce serving of Kraft Shredded Cheese, Mild Cheddar
   100 calories
   8 grams of fat, 6 of them saturated
   30 milligrams of cholesterol
   0 grams of fiber

Winner: Daiya. Fewer calories per serving, lower overall fat content, *dramatically* lower saturated fat, no cholesterol, *and* it contains fiber. (Daiya, by the way, is my favorite brand because it melts so beautifully on pizza dough or on toast; I especially love their mozzarella.)

1 ounce serving of Follow Your Heart Mozzarella Gourmet
    70 calories
    7 grams of fat, 0.5 of it saturated
    0 milligrams of cholesterol (Did you know that cholesterol
        essentially only comes from animal sources? There are
        tiny traces of cholesterol in plants, but the total amount is
        barely measurable.)
    1 gram of fiber

1 ounce serving of whole milk mozzarella
    84 calories
    6 grams of fat, 4 of them saturated
    22 milligrams of cholesterol
    0 grams of fiber

Winner: Follow Your Heart. Lower calories, virtually no saturated fat, no cholesterol, *and* it contains fiber.

One 2-tablespoon serving of Tofutti Plain Cream Cheese (the plain is the nonhydrogenated option)
    85 calories
    5 grams of fat, 2 of them saturated
    0 milligrams of cholesterol
    0 grams of fiber

One 2-tablespoon serving of Kraft Philadelphia Cream Cheese
    100 calories
    9 grams of fat, 6 of them saturated
    30 milligrams of cholesterol
    0 grams of fiber

Winner: Tofutti. It packs 4 fewer grams of fat in the same serving size, plus 4 grams less saturated fat, and absolutely no cholesterol.

And if you were to go with Follow Your Heart Cream Cheese, it has 2 grams of fiber and no trans fats, even though it has more calories and fat. So it, too, is a good alternative.

The American Paradox

Funny thing: with all the low-fat and skim options of milk and cheese we have on the shelves, Americans overall have just gotten fatter. As you'll recall from Day 6, Trade Your Milk and Butter, when you cut down on the fat and opt for skim milk cheese (or skim milk) the milk *sugar* actually increases, which is not good for the waistline. Also, according to a study published in the *Journal of Chromatography*, skim milk actually has more hormones in it than whole milk (not added, mind you, but just in the milk itself), and all those hormones present a big problem for our health. Skim milk has been linked to prostate cancer, and the roughly dozen steroid hormones that can be found in skim milk may increase the odds of ovarian and breast cancer. And of course, hormones are an aggravating factor in acne, too.

Why so many naturally occurring hormones in dairy? Well, just think of it: in order for the mama cow to produce milk, she has to be lactating. When a cow (or a woman) is lactating, her hormones are skyrocketing. As with milk, don't be fooled into thinking that the answer to weight loss is to eat lower-fat or fat-free versions of the dairy cheese you already eat. The past few decades have shown millions of people that this approach isn't at all effective.

If It's Rich, Creamy Mouthfeel You're After: Some Alternatives to the Cheese Alternatives

Of course, there are times when you just want something a little different, and this is where foods with a naturally creamy texture are perfect alternatives. For your tacos, you can use avocados or a little bit of guacamole. Avocados contain fat, but it's the heart- and waist-healthy monounsaturated fat, making them yet another way to get creaminess without all the saturated fats (and again, with the addition of fiber). Avocados do have fat, though, so easy does it!

1-ounce serving of avocado
   47 calories
   4 grams of fat, 1 of them saturated
   0 milligrams of cholesterol
   2 grams of carbohydrates
   2 grams of fiber

Hummus, baba ghanoush, and black bean spreads are also very easy to make at home if you can't find them premade at the grocery, and there are hundreds of ways to flavor them. These internationally inspired foods are enjoying more mainstream popularity, and are now found in virtually any grocery store deli. The velvety taste and texture of bean spreads is even more prominent when they're heated up.

For a quick snack or breakfast, try hummus on a flax cracker. And if you make pizza at home, try using a bean spread in place of the cheese. If you order pizza out, try a local chain instead of one of the national ones; locally owned places are more likely to offer pizzas with bean spreads, and some now offer pizzas topped with Daiya. ZPizza, a chain of fantastic pizza restaurants that has shops in nearly 20 states and counting, offers a vegan pizza with veggie sausage and Daiya, and it's truly to die for. (That's not to say you should have it often, mind you, but rather as a treat! The nondairy cheese still has a lot of fat and salt in it, so keep that in mind as you lean more into whole foods like beans, grains, veggies, and fruits.)

So this is what you will be leaning in with today: wherever you would have had cow or goat cheese, have nondairy cheese instead. You can try any of the brands made from soy, rice, or tapioca, or anything else plant-based; or you can lean a little further into healthy eating by using a bean or avocado spread where you would have used dairy cheese.

So, what are you going to do today?

✓ Drink lots of water.
✓ Eat a hearty breakfast.
✓ Eat an apple.
✓ Just for today, say no to your poison.
✓ Go a little nuts.
✓ Trade up the milk and butter.
✓ Put a little flax on it.
✓ Do a deep dive for five.
✓ Switch up your drinks.
✓ Make lunch without animal products.
✓ Take your vites.
✓ Add in some exercise.
✓ Change up your cheese.

Day 14.

Eat a Superfood

TODAY WE'RE GOING TO LOOK AT SUPERFOODS, WHICH ARE NOT ONLY supernutritious but also super for helping you get in shape, lose weight, and feel vigorous.

I like the word *superfood*. Sounds kind of like a superhero of foods, doesn't it? Well, that's pretty much the case. Superfoods are extremely potent, nutrient-dense foods that can increase the vital force in your body so that you can detoxify, get your immune system to function optimally, and start feeling balanced and energized. They are superconcentrated with disease-fighting phytochemicals and are naturally low in calories. And as tasty and all-around satisfying as they are, they act like medicine in the body, healing you at deep levels and in multiple ways.

The more you work these superheroes into your diet, the more you will simply lose interest in the unhealthier foods you are used to. All of which means your digestion will improve, you'll have the energy to be more active, your cravings will subside, and the weight will continue to come off.

As we've seen, being deficient in vitamins and minerals can create food cravings, the body knows it hasn't gotten what it needs and sends you out for more. By feeding your body nutrient-dense foods, you curb cravings that would otherwise tempt you. So that's the mission today: to discover foods that are brimming with nutrients and medicinal antioxidants.

> **By feeding your body nutrient-dense foods, you curb cravings that would otherwise tempt you.**

Let's look at a few of my favorites so that you can choose which one to work into your plan today.

Goji Berries

Goji berries are a sweet red fruit with a flavor profile that falls somewhere between a cherry and a cranberry. They are tiny little red berries that, when dried, look sort of like skinny raisins. They have been used in Chinese medicine for thousands of years to increase strength, bring about longevity, and enhance sexual energy (see, a bonus!). They contain the highest levels of antioxidants in the world, which means they have the ability to take away the negative effect of free radicals. Free radicals injure cells, cause disease, and promote aging.

Goji berries are low on the glycemic index (which means that they won't send your blood sugar into a tailspin, but more on that soon) and high in fiber, thus making them an excellent snack to keep you feeling balanced and your energy high. Eating the berries will help keep your cravings in check!

But that's not all. Goji berries also have lots of chromium, a mineral that assists the weight loss process. While chromium helps regulate your blood sugar, it also aids in preserving lean muscle mass. Muscles are more efficient at burning calories than fat, so this will keep your metabolism working optimally.

Enjoy a handful of dried goji berries, either by themselves or mixed into a salad or main course. I like to eat them in the morning with my oatmeal or brown rice, so I start out my day supercharged.

Chocolate

The good news of the day (week/month/year)! Chocolate is actually good for you and can be eaten without guilt as part of your weight loss program.

You read that right.

Chocolate is actually good for you and can be eaten without guilt as part of your weight loss program.

Now, what's so great about chocolate? A lot! It's loaded with flavonoids, which increase the elasticity of blood vessels; that's good for the circulation to your heart and brain. It also has tons of antioxidants, which, again, protect us from cell degeneration and disease. Cocoa is also a great source of magnesium, which is good for building strong bones, increasing flexibility, relaxing muscles, and assisting in healthy bowel movements. It has iron in it, which keeps our blood oxygenated; chromium, which, again, helps to balance blood sugar; and zinc, which is critical in keeping the immune system, liver, and pancreas working well. Chocolate also has the same chemical, phenylethylamine (PEA), that your body produces when you are falling in love, so it encourages your brain to produce feel-good endorphins. PEA also helps you to be alert and focused, and along with magnesium, acts as a natural appetite suppressant. And believe it or not, there's lots of fiber in chocolate, so it will help in keeping the intestines clean and bowel movements flowing!

I like chocolate because when I crave a little something sweet, I have a couple of squares (roughly ½ ounce) of a raw, organic chocolate bar and I'm satisfied. I also keep in my fridge a little jar of my favorite Uli Mana dark cacao truffles (*cacao* is another word for chocolate, as is *cocoa*), and have one as a little pick-me-up between meals. It not only curbs the cravings, but it's doing great things for the bod. You might also try a small fistful of cocoa nibs (just the raw cacao beans); eat them as is, or add them into your smoothie or into a trail mix with the goji berries and some nuts. I also buy cocoa powder to add to an occasional peanut butter and banana smoothie—one of my favorites. Talk about heaven!

But let's be clear here: I'm not talking about Snickers bars. I'm talking about cacao, or cocoa, beans—minus all the sugar and dairy you might normally see in chocolate bars.

If you choose to eat chocolate, and I highly recommend that you do, just make sure it's at least 70 percent cocoa and that it's dairy-free. The less sugar it has, the less your blood sugar will zip up and make you hungry for more later on.

I'll be honest with you: if you are used to sweet milk chocolate, there will be a taste bud adjustment when you try the healthier version with no dairy or sugar, but if you don't love it right away, I know you will soon enough. Hey, did you ever think you'd be reading a weight loss book that was encouraging you to keep giving chocolate a try? Yep, I aim to please!

> **Just make sure it's at least 70 percent cocoa and that it's dairy-free.**

My half-sister, Kathy, loves chocolate and worried about having to give it up. She says, "My biggest craving is for chocolate, which is really easy to satisfy with a little bite of super-healthy raw, dark chocolate—the kind that doesn't contain any milk. I make sure I get the kind with absolutely no sugar. It was bitter at first, but I quickly grew to love it. A completely guilt-free pleasure."

Chia Seeds

Chia seeds are an excellent source of antioxidants, omega-3 fatty acids, calcium, and a good source of protein. They don't have much of a taste, are low in saturated fat, and contain no cholesterol. Along with an impressive amount of fiber, which can help lower cholesterol, they also have a good amount of calcium, manganese, thiamine, and phosphorus—vitamins and minerals you might well be lacking in your regular diet.

The word *chia* comes from the Mayan word *chiháan*, which means "strengthening." Native North and South American peoples have historically used chia seeds for endurance.

When you combine chia seeds with liquid (put them into a smoothie, for instance), they soak up the water and form a gel because of the soluble fiber they contain. So drink up fast before you need a spoon!

Chia seeds absorb seven times their weight in water and provide excellent lubrication for the body. This helps you feel full with smaller amounts of food, while also slowing the impact on your blood sugar of the foods that you consume along with the seeds. They help to slow down the absorption of carbohydrates—thus no crashing and craving sugary foods. For instance, because ripe bananas are high on the glycemic index (they act a little like sugar in your body), it's a good idea to throw chia seeds into a shake if you have bananas in the mix (more on the glycemic index on Day 26). Chia seeds have long been used to correct constipation; they act like a scrub brush that cleans out your intestines as they move through your digestive system.

To get the greatest health benefits, consume chia seeds in their whole state (grinding them is fine, as that retains all the fiber and nutrients as well) rather than as an oil or supplement. Aside from putting them in a smoothie, you can also sprinkle them atop your oatmeal along with some chopped fruit, or mix them into a soy or rice yogurt, or add them as texture to a salad, or as thickener to a pasta sauce.

As with any nuts or seeds, chias are calorie dense, so stick to around a tablespoon. The high nutritional value of chia seeds will give you a more robust level of energy, enabling you to expend that energy on a good hike or run, all the while keeping hunger pangs at bay.

You can usually find them at your local grocery, but if not, do a search online and order them.

Extra Lean: If your blood sugar tends to rise after eating fruit (mine doesn't; it varies from person to person, though), try eating a few nuts first, about 25 minutes beforehand. Also, stick to whole raw fruit rather than cooked, dried, or extra ripe.

Blueberries

Blueberries are so common and popular you might overlook just how powerful they are in terms of their health-giving properties. As with all the superfoods, blueberries are full of antioxidants—more than most other fruits and vegetables even—to combat inflammation, disease, and aging. They have multiple phytonutrients and phytoflavonoids, which are supportive to the nervous system, brain, cardiovascular system, and contain a good amount of vitamin C, vitamin E, potassium, manganese, and of course our favorite—fiber.

They also have something called ellagic acid in them, an antioxidant that is said to reduce the risk of cancer by blocking metabolic pathways that lead to cancer. Studies show that the anthocyanin pigments in the berries may actually halt cancer in the critical stages of promotion and proliferation, and ellagic acid may also slow the growth of some cancerous tumors.

Blueberries are a nutritional powerhouse without a lot of calories. They have no fat or cholesterol, and are excellent for your digestion and for avoiding constipation, thus protecting your colon from disease. When you are losing weight, or anytime really, it's important to keep eliminating the waste and detoxing your body naturally. The natural tannins in berries reduce inflammation in the digestive tract, which will help you feel clean and slim.

Blueberries are an excellent snack or an addition to breakfast oatmeal or rice; you can throw them into a smoothie, or have them for dessert with a little nondairy milk poured on top. They are low on the glycemic index, so again, they will keep you feeling steady, fulfilled, and free from cravings. In fact, research shows that people with type 2 diabetes, insulin resistance, or metabolic syndrome do well by eating blueberries, as they have a favorable influence on blood sugar regulation. If you choose blueberries as your superfood for the day (and you can certainly choose to have the other super-foods, as well), have at least a cup either fresh or frozen.

Kale

Okay, everything so far has been easy to love. Nutty, fruity, choco-laty flavors are certainly delightful to incorporate into your day. But I can't let you go before talking about the most powerful green on the planet—kale.

If you aren't familiar with it, let me make the introduction. Kale is that frilly deep green stuff that you often see as the garnish in a steakhouse, which is crazy since it should really be front and cen-ter on your plate. As with all our food superheroes, kale is high in fiber, and will go far to fill you up and keep you feeling full; and as it works its way out of your bod, it'll clean out all the gunk that's in your colon. It's a member of the cruciferous family of vegetables, and it's extremely rich in nutrients, including vitamins A, C, K, calcium, folic acid, as well as all those miraculous antioxidants. It helps to lower your cholesterol by binding with the bile acids in your diges-tive tract, and then gets excreted along with them.

Kale is said to be an excellent anticancer food, protecting against breast, prostate, colon, ovarian, and bladder cancer, specifi-cally. The abundant flavonoids in kale have an anti-inflammatory effect, which calms the body and protects it from chronic or degen-erative disease.

You can steam or sauté it in a tiny bit of olive oil or orange juice; you can add it to soups or stir-fries. You can mix it into pasta or sneak it onto a sandwich. My favorite way of enjoying kale is to juice it, but more on that in our fourth week, on Day 25. Friends of mine love kale "chips"—torn-up leaves tossed in just a tiny bit of olive oil and roasted in the oven at 300 degrees for 20 minutes to a half hour (check every 5 to 10 minutes and turn as necessary). Some people like to sprinkle a little nutritional yeast on the kale before or after roasting. (Not to be confused with the kind of yeast you use in bread or beer, nutritional yeast is a yellow flake or powder that has a wonderful cheesy taste. You'll find it at any natural foods store.) Kids *love* kale chips, too.

If I had to pick the most powerful superfood that does the most good in the body, kale would be it.

So there you have a short list of superfoods to choose from. Make sure you have at least one of these today and every day you are on the Lean plan. You

If I had to pick the most powerful superfood that would do the most good in the body, kale would be it.

can have all of them on a single day, too, so feel free to work them all in. Remember, this is not about dieting, but rather creating a way of eating that crowds out hunger and leaves little to no room to indulge in the old bad habits. The more you tuck into these nutrient-dense, fiber-rich foods, the less you will have a hankering for burgers and fries. These superfoods act like medicine in your body, helping you to detox years of bad choices. They will help clean your cells and have everything working optimally, so that you feel better and become more active, more attuned to healthy choices.

So, what are you going to do today?

- ✓ Drink lots of water.
- ✓ Eat a hearty breakfast.
- ✓ Eat an apple.
- ✓ Just for today, say no to your poison.
- ✓ Go a little nuts.
- ✓ Trade up the milk and butter.
- ✓ Put a little flax on it.
- ✓ Do a deep dive for five.
- ✓ Switch up your drinks.

✓ Make lunch without animal products.
✓ Take your vites.
✓ Add in some exercise.
✓ Change up your cheese.
✓ Eat a superfood.

Day 15.

Love Yourself a Little

Two weeks down and two to go. Today we're going to take another break from food talk. I know you're drinking your water, eating your hearty breakfast, eating lots of powerfoods, and generally staying away from animal-derived foods, at least at breakfast and lunch. Today all I want you to do is find some time to be kind to yourself.

Before you start rolling your eyes and muttering "Puleeze," listen up, because I'm serious. You can't expect to achieve lasting weight loss results if you don't regard yourself with kindness. Because those little bits of self-loathing or unkindness that sneak up on us are what lead us to the cookie jar or the snack bin.

I'm talking about loving yourself as well as you love everyone else. Or even better. Right now. Just as you are.

It doesn't matter what the number is on the scale, or how your clothes fit, or how well (or not) you've stuck to the plan. Your task for today is to throw yourself a little tenderness, a little fondness.

I'm going to show you exactly how to do it in a very methodical way that wont take long at all, so it's not like you'll be going into deep therapy. This will take you about a minute to do, and if you do it three times today, you will begin to feel different very soon.

But first, let's look more closely at why this tweak is even necessary.

Here's the thing: if you are struggling with your weight, you likely get irritated or even ashamed of yourself for not having it together better. You may think you are weak-willed or flawed in character because you can't seem to make yourself look like you think you should. You look in the mirror and scan your body and feel deep disappointment. You may even think you are, at your core, repugnant and unlovable. If I've heard it once I've heard it a hundred times: "I feel so bad about myself I end up deciding, why not just eat whatever I want? I look terrible anyway, so what difference does it make?" Do you see how the cycle of self-hatred perpetuates the weight problem? If you don't feel affection for yourself, why would you make choices that actually benefit yourself?

Feeling bad about yourself, though, didn't start with your not having the ideal body. I can almost guarantee you that. It likely had its roots in something else.

Let's go back in time a bit, back to when you were just a kid. Since few of us had perfect childhoods, I think it's safe to say that at some point someone made us feel profoundly bad about who we were. It could have been a parent, someone(s) in our social group, the culture, or a teacher. But somewhere along the line early on, we were told (and told in such a way that it cut to the bone and made an impact) that there was a part of us that was not okay or right. And that whatever was "not okay" about us had better cease to be. In other words, if we ever wanted to be liked or accepted, we'd better get rid of that part of us that was unlikable and never let it see the light of day again.

For me, I learned that being needy (wanting to be held or told that I am wonderful) was annoying and made people go away. I also learned that being silly or playful was distasteful and made me unlikable. Being confident and wanting to perform was perceived as arrogance and being full of myself. So those three qualities—neediness, silliness, and confidence—make up my personal "shadow."

Your shadow is unique to you, and it can shift and change a bit with new experiences. The shadow, and everyone has one, is an accumulation of qualities that we were told make us repellent, unlovable, unacceptable. It's the shadow that's the basis of our self-loathing.

> **Extra Lean:** Get a massage or ask a loved one to rub your shoulders and feet; sometimes we seek comfort in food when touch would really do the trick better. Seek love, not food!

Carl Jung introduced the idea of the shadow as an archetype (a pattern of thought that exists in all of us); he described it as our dark side, the unconscious part of us that houses all the raw thoughts and desires we are ashamed to admit to. This part of our psyche contains those aspects of our character that—again, thanks to a disapproving society, shaming parent, or strict religious ethos—we cannot acknowledge or act out. He says that when we were very young we received the message that these traits were bad, and we repressed or denied them. To our conscious mind, these inadmissible parts of our self ceased to exist. In their place we developed a mask, a more pleasing and acceptable front to present to the world.

In *A Little Book on the Human Shadow,* the poet Robert Bly elaborated on this theme by saying that we were all born with a personality that expressed the entirety of our human nature without restriction. As we grew up, we were taught that certain parts of ourselves (sexuality, confidence, anger, impishness) were deplorable. So somewhere deep inside we made a decision not to be that way anymore. Bly says it was as if we stuffed into a bag all those undesirable pieces of ourselves, and then we had to lug the bag around—hidden—for the rest of our lives. In therapeutic terms, we *disowned* a significant part of who we are.

Jung tells us that once we reintegrate the shadow, we can use all those suppressed aspects to unlock our creativity and to access our higher Self. And by tapping into our higher Self, all things become possible. By making peace with what we thought was so ugly in us, we bring peace to our lives; and I would say that by going further and actually loving that shadow we can begin to make healthy choices that reflect the kindness we feel for ourselves.

And this is the surprising thing: our shadow is actually the most spirited, pure part of ourselves, the part that actually holds the magic. It is our vulnerability and truth, the part we turned away from to go out and face the world with a carefully constructed façade. But a façade is just that, it's a false self; and because it's a false self, a sort of mask, our unacknowledged shadow prevents us from having all our power and thrust to really live fully and take care of ourselves.

So when we get back in touch with our shadow and come to love it, we become more "whole," more integrated. We don't abhor a part of ourselves and thus act out in ways that are unloving (eating bad food which makes us fat and unhealthy, for instance).

Go grab a pen and paper or your computer.

Make a list of three things you consider a part of your shadow self. Now direct some loving thoughts or words at each of those things. Example: You've heard three of the things I struggle with, so I would say to the "needy" part of me: "You aren't needy, dearest. You crave connection and you want to see and be seen. Smart gal (or fella). Pity you didn't get it back then, but I'm glad you're someone in your adult life who is comfortable reaching out for love." I'd say to the "silly" part of me that I once shunned: "Oh man, are you wild and free; how awesome!" See how easy it is to turn things around? And trust me, before you know it, you'll actually start believing this stuff!

Now write down three things you love about yourself. And if you can't think of three, think about what other people love about you and write down whatever comes to mind.

Some examples: I am a kind person. I recognize a truth when

I hear it, and am not lazy about moving on it. I speak out when I see someone getting mistreated. I care about my co-workers. I am funny.

Now read your list out loud.

The first time you do this, it might take ten minutes or so just to write down the three things. But soon you'll be able to conjure them up quickly, in thirty seconds even. Look back at the list several times today, and then a few times a day in the following days, so that you are checking in regularly and loving up your shadow.

Remember, your shadow is part of you, and like Jung implied, it's actually the key to your mojo (okay, so he didn't use *that* word). It's the most real and genuine part of yourself, so to really move forward in your life—with weight loss, romance, success, or anything—you have to feel an inward goodwill. When you do, everything else will follow. You will feed yourself in a way that is loving, take care of your body in a way that is loving, and surround yourself with people who are supportive and loving. It all starts with you, so close your eyes, and keep checking in!

Whenever you feel tempted throughout the day to curse or shame yourself, remember the one inside whom you are hurting. Stop yourself—or shield yourself from someone who wants to hurt you— and redirect your sentiments to kindness and compassion.

So, what are you going to do today?

- ✓ Drink lots of water.
- ✓ Eat a hearty breakfast.
- ✓ Eat an apple.
- ✓ Just for today, say no to your poison.
- ✓ Go a little nuts.
- ✓ Trade up the milk and butter.
- ✓ Put a little flax on it.
- ✓ Do a deep dive for five.
- ✓ Switch up your drinks.
- ✓ Make lunch without animal products.

✓ Take your vites.
✓ Add in some exercise.
✓ Change up your cheese.
✓ Eat a superfood.
✓ Love yourself a little.

DAY 16.

Toss Up a Big Bowl of Love, a.k.a. Salad

TODAY, YOUR LEAN IS GREEN. AND RED. AND DELICIOUS.

As you've seen already in these first few days, the Lean is mostly about *adding* new things to your daily routine. Sure, some days you'll also be removing things like milk or meat, but mostly I want to show you how *adding* things like lots of clean water or a big bowl of oatmeal is the way toward a better body. Because what you *include* in your diet is just as important as what you *exclude*.

Today is an add day—a very yummy add day. All I want you to do is make yourself a nice big salad. I like to call it the Big Bowl of Love, because this salad has so much fiber, nutrition, and fabulous energizing food that I sort of see it as a lip-smacking present we can bestow on our precious bods. And trust me, your bod will thank you.

By the way, when I say big salad, I mean BIG. Not just a little side dish of lettuce and tomatoes, but a big mixing bowl's worth of just about everything you can fit in. I want you to make your salad as colorful as you can because the more color you have in your bowl, the more diversity of nutrients you'll be consuming. Throw in a few things that are varying shades of red, green, and orange, and have a bunch of different textures so that every bite is a flavor and mouthfeel sensation. Make enough for whoever will be joining you at the table, because after all, don't you want to share the love?

I want you to make six cups of salad or more. You may sometimes find this to be a meal in itself, especially on warm days, but it doesn't have to be. It can be a snack, a side, or the main event. You can have it whenever you want during the day, and you can split it up and have a little a couple of times a day, but by day's end, you must finish the salad. Why?

Adding a salad to your daily meal plan is a great weight loss strategy and fits right in to our "crowding out" approach. It fills you up with good roughage—lettuces, veggies, fruits, and seeds are all full of healthy fiber—thereby leaving less room in the belly for over-stuffing yourself. It allows you to feel fuller while eating fewer total calories because all that miraculous fiber is busy absorbing water and bulking up in your stomach. And did I mention fiber itself has no calories at all? That's right, no calories, and it crowds out the junk. It's far better to curb your appetite with some bright orange carrots or rippled red radishes than with some chips and dip or a side of fries. You'll feel so loved with all that fresh food pouring pure nourishment into your bloodstream, you'll know your doing your body a mitzvah.

But it's not just the fiber that you benefit from; you are also scoring all the good nutrition that comes along with eating raw goodies that are grown in the ground or on trees. This big bowl of fresh food is sort of one-stop shopping for vitamin C, E, A, beta-carotene, and a whole host of powerful antioxidants. There is practically no nutrient you can't get from a plentiful salad. As a matter of fact, if put together thoughtfully with a wide variety of veggies and fruits, your salad will be much more of a complete meal than a lot of other food possibilities you might be used to. And remember, your gut has sensors that tell the brain when it has the nutrition it needs, and when the needs are met, the "go get more food" message is turned off.

You are going to use beans, legumes, or seeds (sometimes all of them!) in your salad too, so you will be enjoying lots of protein along with the fiber and minerals. No animal gunk like chicken or cow's milk cheese in this gorgeous bowl, please; just keep it lively with the stuff grown in nature. It doesn't take much of things like toasted pumpkin seeds or raw walnuts to add some trace minerals to the ultimate nutrient equation, so enjoy your salad, knowing it's going to work wonders in every single cell of your being.

> **Extra Lean:** There is no nutritional difference between dried or canned beans, but since canned can be high in sodium, rinse and drain before use.

Salad is also an excellent plate filler and will make all your meals look more abundant and attractive. For instance, if you are having some pasta for dinner, and you put a big mound of salad on your dish alongside the spaghetti, the serving size of pasta will have to be small enough to make room for the salad.

I always love mixing together pasta or casserole or whatever is on the menu on the same forkful with some crunchy veggies. Every bite is hearty that way!

If you can hit a farmers' market, that's ideal; but a good grocery store (make a road trip if you don't have one in your neighborhood) will carry everything you need. Try to buy what's in season, and if you can spring for organic, do it. Start with some nutrient-rich lettuces like romaine or a spring mix; I also like to add some arugula or spinach. Avoid iceberg lettuce—it's the least nutritious of them all. From there, add in a selection of leafy greens, root vegetables, berries, and seeds. Use your imagination and try different things, rotating the mix as you get bored or see new produce you'd like to try.

It's best if you can buy and mix all the ingredients yourself, but if you are in a hurry and are visiting a salad bar, just be sure to steer clear of premade mixes like bean salads (they are often laden with fattening oils), croutons, or chunks of cheese, and just stick to completely whole foods that aren't processed. It's okay to have some processed foods sometimes, but let's keep this Big Bowl of Love pure and simple. Here are some other ingredients I like to toss in, but bear in mind that you can change it up according to your tastes and desires!

- any kind or mix of lettuces
- red cabbage
- carrot
- cucumber
- a small handful of toasted pumpkin seeds
- crushed raw walnuts
- sun-dried, thinly sliced figs
- chickpeas
- broccoli or cauliflower (raw or steamed and chilled)
- red, green, or orange bell pepper
- celery
- avocado
- sweet Vidalia onions
- red onions
- radish
- cubed tofu or tempeh
- blueberries, raspberries, blackberries
- chopped or sliced apple or pear
- hearts of palm
- roasted red pepper
- black beans or any kind of bean
- sunflower seeds
- chia seeds
- artichoke hearts

Extra Lean: If you feel gassy when eating beans or certain vegetables, cook them really well next time so that they are soft and easier to digest. And try some Beano or digestive enzymes to help while your body adjusts to all the fiber. (Your body *will* adjust, I promise!)

Chop everything into bite-size pieces. Mix and match any or all of the above ingredients. Use a salad dressing that is nondairy and not too heavy. (The recipe for my favorite dressing—vegan ranch—is in the recipe section.)

Enjoy, and know that your body is being seriously loved up by this one!

So, what are you going to do today?

✓ Drink lots of water.
✓ Eat a hearty breakfast.
✓ Eat an apple.
✓ Just for today, say no to your poison.
✓ Go a little nuts.
✓ Trade up the milk and butter.
✓ Put a little flax on it.
✓ Do a deep dive for five.
✓ Switch up your drinks.
✓ Make lunch without animal products.
✓ Take your vites.
✓ Add in some exercise.
✓ Change up your cheese.
✓ Eat a superfood.
✓ Love yourself a little.
✓ Toss up a big bowl of salad.

DAY 17.

Make Some Cashew Cream

IT'S DAY 17. TODAY, WE'RE GOING WITH OPTIONS—YOUR FIRST DAY where, if you prefer, you can skip it. But I think you'll like this one. Because if you are someone who, like me, finds it hard to live without the luxury of creaminess in a dish here or there, I think this might just be a perfect solution for you!

I love everything creamy. I love cream sauces, cream-based soups, and cream poured over desserts. The texture of cream is comforting and luxurious, and it makes me feel full and indulged and happy. Trust me, the happiness lasts longer when there is no guilt following closely behind. The cream I'm going to introduce to you today is not made from dairy. There is not an ounce of cholesterol in it, and it's actually quite healthy. Kind of magic sounding, no?

Well, we have my friend Tal Ronnen to thank for this elixir of deliciousness. Tal is a vegan chef—one of the best and certainly the most recognized in the world. He was classically trained to cook using French culinary techniques, and since dairy cream has a good hand in many of those techniques, he had to figure out something else to use since the heavy stuff was so problematic (fattening and artery clogging . . . plus Tal had a sweet spot for dairy cows and didn't think it right to take their milk!). So he took a cue from the raw food movement. Raw foodies had been using cashew cream for decades to add texture to desserts and sauces. But raw foodies, as you may know, don't cook with heat above 104 or 118 degrees Fahrenheit (it varies depending on who you are talking to).

Tal realized that actually cooking with cashew cream was even more beneficial and exciting than using it cold because it reduces and thickens like heavy cream. He uses it for sauces, soups, or to add a rich creamy texture to things like mashed potatoes.

Tal said cashew cream "definitely changed how I cook. I was never able to make those thick, creamy sauces with other nondairy milks, like soy or rice milk. They have very little fat in them, so I'd put them in a pan over high heat, and they would just evaporate instead of reducing like heavy cream does."

I'm including what sems like an indulgence in the Lean plan because I really do think cashew cream is one of the magic ingredients that makes it so easy to live without dairy. You can use it as an Alfredo sauce or as a base for a quick homespun pudding (add a little agave to it) to drizzle over cooked fruit. You can store it for two to three days in the fridge, or you can freeze it for up to six months and then thaw it out as needed. (Tal warns that it can be a bit lumpy after being frozen, but a spin in the blender will smooth it out nicely.) You see, the Lean is not about being deprived; you are just crowding out the bad stuff with a really good alternative.

Here's Tal, explaining how to use it.

> **Cashew cream is one of the magic ingredients that makes it so easy to live without dairy. You can use it as an Alfredo sauce or as a base for a quick homespun pudding (add a little agave to it) to drizzle over cooked fruit.**

The trick when making cashew cream is to use raw cashews. They have no flavor of their own; they're just a vessel for fat and creaminess. (It's the roasting that brings out the familiar sweetness in cashews.) Because it has a nice fat content, cashew cream reduces in a pan even faster than heavy cream.

For different applications, there are different consistencies— thick and regular. Both are easy to make but not quick because the cashews need to soak overnight. A shortcut is to put the cashews in a pot with water, bring them to a boil, then shut off the heat and let them soak for an hour. But this starts to leach out the sweetness, so you're better off with the overnight method. Also, there's at least one decent brand of store-bought nut cream, called MimicCreme, which combines cashews and almonds; you can usually find it on the shelves or in the refrigerated section near the soy milk. Of course, nothing compares to homemade, and once you get used to it, there may be no turning back.

REGULAR AND THICK CASHEW CREAM

Makes about 2¼ cups thick cream or 3½ cups regular cream
Active time: 5–10 minutes
Start to finish: About 12 hours

> 2 cups whole raw cashews (not pieces, which are often
>   dry), rinsed very well under cold water

1. Put the cashews in a bowl and add cold water to cover them. Cover the bowl and refrigerate overnight.
2. Drain the cashews and rinse under cold water. Place them in a blender with enough fresh cold water to cover them by 1 inch. Blend on high for several minutes until very smooth. (If you're not using a professional high-speed blender such as a Vitamix, which creates an ultra-smooth cream, strain the cashew cream through a fine-mesh sieve.)
3. To make a thicker cashew cream, simply reduce the amount of water in the initial blend, so that the water just slightly covers the cashews.

In the back of this book, there are some wonderful recipes for soups and a main course using the cream; and there is also a wonderful apple crumble over which you can drizzle the cashew cream for an even more delicious final touch.

Now, all of this said, I want to remind you that cashew cream does have fat in it, so it's not something you want to use every day. This tweak is so that you don't feel deprived, so that you see there is really nothing you can't replace and make healthier. *Sigh*. I'm so glad Tal figured this one out because creaminess is one of life's little pleasures!

So, what are you going to do today?

✓ Drink lots of water.
✓ Eat a hearty breakfast.
✓ Eat an apple.
✓ Just for today, say no to your poison.
✓ Go a little nuts.
✓ Trade up the milk and butter.
✓ Put a little flax on it.
✓ Do a deep dive for five.
✓ Switch up your drinks.
✓ Make lunch without animal products.
✓ Take your vites.
✓ Add in some exercise.
✓ Change up your cheese.
✓ Eat a superfood.
✓ Love yourself a little.
✓ Toss up a big bowl of salad.
✓ Make some cashew cream (if it's creaminess you need).

Day 18.

Take the Animals off the Dinner Plate

Big lean today! You might even call it a leap. Today I want you to take the animals—and anything that comes from them, like eggs or cheese—off your dinner plate.

You've been getting some practice with breakfast and lunch, and you've even learned to crowd out your snacks—by eating a superfood or opting for nuts, for instance—so that they are free of animal stuff, too. Bravo, you! Now we are going to lean a little further toward weight loss and health by eating some delicious food that, unlike all animal foods, has zero cholesterol. And lots of nutrients. And in the process we're going to rev up your metabolism and cut out more of the problematic fat.

I know. You may be thinking, *Hang on a minute, you can't just take away all my favorite foods one by one.*

I wouldn't dream of it.

I, too, grew up loving barbecue chicken, burgers, and pasta with sausage. If you had told me back when I was twenty that I had to have even one meal without meat I would have protested (well, unless the meal was popcorn and soda while watching a movie!). And I might have even panicked a little. But I won't leave you at a loss, I promise, and there is no need to panic. I've got some good solutions for you to make this move a smooth one. But before I tell you what you *will* be eating, let's talk a little about protein, since most people equate protein with animal foods or are just confused about how much and what types of protein they really need.

What Protein Is and Why It's Important for Weight Loss

Proteins are one of the essential building blocks of your body. Basically, they're what we're made of, and they are vital to the body's continued functioning. Proteins are macronutrients composed of 20 amino acids, connected and folded into various chains; the amounts and combinations of these amino acid chains determine what kind of protein they make. Everything that you are is made of, with, and by proteins—muscles, organs, the lenses of your eyes—right down to your fingernails. So what does protein have to do with weight loss?

Protein enhances weight loss in three ways. One is appetite reduction. Researchers believe that protein makes you feel more satiated than fats or carbohydrates, thereby curbing your appetite and decreasing your overall calorie intake. Increased protein in a meal triggers the production of hormones that signal your brain that you're full.

The best way to game your body into feeling fuller at each meal is by ensuring that you're eating enough of the right kinds of protein. This doesn't mean so-called lean meats like chicken, turkey, or low-fat cheese, which even in their "lean" version still contain large amounts of heart-damaging saturated fats. It means incorporating greater amounts of the higher-quality proteins found in beans, legumes, soy foods like tempeh or tofu, and seitan (a wheat-based meat replacement). Eating the right amount of foods makes it entirely possible to lose weight *and* avoid the constipation and bad breath associated with high-fat, low-fiber, animal protein–based diets.

A second way good-quality plant protein helps is that it has a high thermic effect (calories burned as body heat during digestion), which amps up your metabolism. According to the Physicians Committee for Responsible Medicine: "Within a few weeks of skipping meat and opting for plant protein, your after-meal metabolism increases so that it is 16 percent faster for around three hours after every meal of nutrient dense, high-fiber protein than with the Standard American Diet of meat and dairy." So when you eat food that is grown in the ground or on trees, you are literally stoking your metabolism. Protein is more effective than other macronutrients like carbohydrates or fat at raising your resting energy-burning level.

Within a few weeks of skipping meat and opting for plant protein, your after-meal metabolism increases.

Protein's third great weight loss benefit is that it makes it easier for your body to hold onto its lean muscle mass while reducing your overall percentage of body fat. So what does that mean? To begin with, lean muscle mass is simply the amount of your body weight that's made up of muscle as opposed to fat (it's very important to remember that *some* body fat is essential—the goal isn't zero).

> **Extra Lean:** Finish eating for the day by 7 p.m. That way you can digest and sleep well, without a full belly. Keeping to this rule will also stop you from late-night grazing.

If you aren't eating an adequate amount of protein while losing weight, you will shed pounds, but you're likely to lose some muscle as well. Muscle mass is smaller than fat, resulting in a slimmer physique, and muscle is also slightly more calorically active than fat. So we want to make sure you are eating enough protein, while reducing fat (which you do automatically when you avoid animal foods) and therefore retaining the muscle.

How Much?

While researching this subject, I've learned that some studies say you need to get 30 percent of your calories from protein to ensure weight loss, while others say it's closer to 15 percent, and Dr. Neal Barnard and others say 10 percent is just perfect. When I asked him what he thought about the whole protein/weight loss thing, he said, "If you look at populations that are thinnest and healthiest, the diet is around 10 percent protein. Foods vary a lot. Broccoli is about 30 percent protein, as a percentage of calories. But satiety claims have been made for protein, for fat, and for carbohydrate, and the only thing I've seen that really bears out is fiber. The more fiber, the fewer calories it takes to be full."

I think the point here is that people are different, and you need simply to make sure to always add in some good plant-based protein to your meals and snacks, whether it's beans or tofu, veggie sausage or hummus. As I mentioned earlier, I don't think we need be mathematicians constantly calculating what the molecular makeup of our food is. That's exhausting, and I think there are more important things to do with our minds. Just note what makes you feel strong and satiated, and that will cue you as to what works for you.

The important thing is that you don't go for animal foods to get your protein, because there are too many problems that go along with eating meat and dairy, and we want you to be smart about your choices. Great sources of protein include seitan, tempeh, beans, lentils, tofu, and the many products made from them. Think black bean chili or scrambled tofu and veggies, alongside a nice big salad or a baked sweet potato. If you are fairly athletic, you might need more—perhaps as much as 1.7 grams per kilogram of body weight.

Great sources of protein include seitan, tempeh, beans, lentils, tofu, and the many products made from them.

Smart Sources

It's more than possible to obtain the protein you need to lose weight from smarter protein sources. Smarter sources contain high amounts of protein, without the artery-clogging fat or cholesterol counts in meat, chicken, and dairy. One of Dr. Walter Willett's top three healthy eating guidelines (he's the chair of the Department of Nutrition at Harvard's School of Public Health) is that we should "emphasize plant sources of protein rather than animal sources."

Keep it simple and just incorporate a fist-size portion of plant protein at every meal.

Keep it simple and just incorporate a fist-size portion of plant protein at every meal. Here are some examples, but bear in mind that you don't need to weigh or calculate; I just want to show you some numbers so you feel good about what you are doing!

*One 4-ounce serving of seitan (sometimes known as wheat meat)**

    120 calories
    2 grams of fat, none of it saturated
    0 milligrams of cholesterol
    0 grams of fiber
    18–26 grams of protein

    * Seitan products are diverse, and have a range of nutritional profiles; additionally, seitan is often made at home. Thus, numbers presented are estimates. Seitan made with whole wheat flour would contain fiber, for example.

One 4-ounce serving of tempeh

    230 calories
    18 grams of fat, 3 of them saturated
    0 milligrams of cholesterol

11 grams of fiber
20 grams of protein

1 cup of quinoa, cooked
222 calories
4 grams of fat, none of it saturated
0 milligrams of cholesterol
5 grams of fiber
8 grams of protein

One 4-ounce serving of tofu
138 calories
8 grams of fat, 1 gram of it saturated
0 milligrams of cholesterol
2 grams of fiber
14 grams of protein

1 cup of lentils, cooked, no salt
230 calories
1 gram of fat, unsaturated
0 milligrams of cholesterol
16 grams of fiber
18 grams of protein

1 ounce serving of almonds, salted, dry roasted
169 calories
15 grams of fat, 1 of them saturated
0 milligrams of cholesterol
3 grams of fiber
6 grams of protein

1 cup of broccoli
54 calories
0 grams of fat

0 milligrams of cholesterol
6 grams of fiber
4 grams of protein

One 4-ounce serving of peas
128 calories
0 grams of fat
0 milligrams of cholesterol
8 grams of fiber
8 grams of protein

Seitan, tempeh, nuts quinoa, tofu, lentils, almonds, broccoli, peas . . . as you can see, protein is found in just about everything that grows in nature. Determining how to obtain enough protein from nonmeat sources isn't difficult; in fact it would be far more complicated to determine which foods *don't* have it! A note here: Did you know that 1 egg has only about 6 grams of protein in it, 2.7 in the yolk and 3.6 in the white? So if you are just eating the white (all that bad cholesterol is in the yolk, after all), you are not getting very much protein at *all*! You get 18 grams of protein in a cup of lentils, plus all that fiber, which is far more satisfying!

The Truth about Protein Combination

Contrary to popular (outdated) belief, a plant-based diet does not require careful combination of specific foods to form "complete" proteins. The body requires 20 amino acids to make all its necessary proteins and optimally carry out its physiological processes; the body produces 11 of them on its own, and the remaining 9 must be obtained from food sources. The "incomplete protein theory" popularized in the late 1970s was based on the premise that the 9 food-sourced amino acids could be acquired only by including meat and dairy foods in the diet. Therefore, the reasoning went, plant-based protein sources were inferior, and getting all 9 amino acids from plant sources required combining foods like rice and beans at each meal.

This belief, popularized back in the 1970s by Frances Moore Lappé, in her otherwise brilliant *Diet for a Small Planet,* has been widely debunked. Lappé herself was simply misinformed and has since recanted her protein combination theory. Since 1993, the American Dietetic Association's position on plant protein has been clear:

> *Plant sources of protein alone can provide adequate amounts of the essential and nonessential amino acids,* assuming that dietary protein sources from plants are reasonably varied and that caloric intake is sufficient to meet energy needs. . . . Conscious combining of these foods within a given meal, as the complementary protein dictum suggests, is unnecessary. (emphasis added)

This simply means you should eat a bunch of different things throughout the day! Keep it varied. Any diet, plant-based or otherwise, is inferior if it isn't varied enough. Food combining isn't necessary, so don't wear yourself out trying to match grains with legumes Instead, focus on expanding the variety and quality of the foods you include in your diet. Nothing makes this easier than crowding the fat and cholesterol sources off your plate and replacing them with superior-quality plant proteins.

Here's Natala again:

> *For dinner I might make an all-veggie lasagna, using white beans to make "ricotta" and a homemade tomato sauce loaded with vegetables, maybe topped off with a few pine nuts. The color of my meals and the quantity makes the change a lot easier than if I were to look for the same exact taste as things I liked before. Now it is about finding all of the foods I've missed out on for so long.*

Okay, so we know what the whole foods look like—veggies, lentils, black beans, quinoa, and the like; but what about things like veggie sausage or "faux" chicken? I *love* them. I love them because I can use these meat alternatives just as I used meat, and they are so much healthier. I wish that we lived in a world where we all had the time, know-how, means, and motivation to prepare healthful, from-scratch meals brimming with organic vegetables, whole grains, and slow-cooked beans; and the movement in that direction is important. There is no doubt that this is the ideal and that we'd all be a lot better off if we ate this way.

But we don't live in a perfect world. And the vast majority of us are surviving on frozen pepperoni pizzas, buckets of chicken, and fast-food burgers. The closest many kids may get to eating a vegetable on any given day may be the french fries on their lunch tray. Plus, some of us have partners who simply love the old "meat and potatoes"–style plate, and simple beans and grains just won't go over, at least not right away. That's why my approach is to take your current lifestyle and eating habits into account, and ease you into eating healthier by showing how easy it is to swap out fattening, high-cholesterol animal products for vegan versions of your traditional favorite foods. I want you to still enjoy your favorite comfort foods; I want you to feel comfortable and excited about changing the way you eat. If you ease yourself away from animal foods by turning to high-protein meat alternatives, you will feel no sacrifice. I think one of the biggest barriers to healthy eating is the emotional bond we have with our traditional foods; we don't want to give them up.

We don't want to live like monks. (Not me, that's for sure!) So although you might hear some healthy people saying they don't like to eat "faux meats," know that you are easing yourself into a new way of eating, and it's just fine. It's infinitely better for you to have veggie sausage than pork or chicken sausage, so much more helpful to weight loss to enjoy plant-based turkey rather than animal turkey. Once the mind opens, it continues to expand, and changing the way we eat is a process. For many people, starting out on transitional foods like vegan meats and cheeses is a first, fantastic step, and they'll likely later incorporate more "real foods" like unprocessed grains, beans, vegetables, and fruits into their diet.

I asked Dr. Michael Greger for his medical opinion on meat alternatives, and this is what he said . . .

KF. How is eating high-protein meat alternatives instead of meat effective for weight loss? Are those veggie substitutes a good idea?

MG. There appears to be something in meat that causes more weight gain than its calorie content would suggest. A study published last year in the world's most prestigious nutrition journal entitled "Meat Consumption and Prospective Weight Change in Participants of the EPIC-PANACEA Study" followed hundreds of thousands of men and women for five years to see which foods were most associated with weight gain.

> **There appears to be something in meat that causes more weight gain than its calorie content would suggest.**

They found that "Total meat consumption was positively associated with weight gain in men and women, in normal-weight and overweight subjects, and in smokers and nonsmokers." They concluded: "Our results suggest that a decrease in meat consumption may improve weight management." And this was after adjusting for initial weight, physical activity, educational level, smoking status, and, ready for the kicker? They controlled for total energy [caloric] intake. So this was after controlling for calories.

One would assume that sure, meat is associated with weight gain because it's so calorically dense, and so you'd just get more calories in your diet compared to those eating vegetarian, for example. But no, this is after controlling for caloric intake. Meaning if there are two people eating the same amount of calories and one person eats more meat than the other—the meat eater gains more weight.

Processed meat was more fattening than red meat, but surprisingly, "The strongest relation with annual weight change was observed for poultry." The shocking conclusion: even if one were to eat the same number of calories of a plant-based meat substitute, one would gain less weight.

So tonight for dinner, have some chik'n Parmesan with rice and green beans. Or a quinoa-based pasta with cashew cream sauce and veggie sausage. Or if it's taco night, use some meatless meat crumbles (find them in your grocer's freezer section) instead of ground beef with a nice big salad. Go to the recipes in the back of this book, and see if you can't find a traditional favorite of yours, just with the animals left off the plate. I think you might be pleased with how it tastes, and your body will feel so good and clean without all the saturated fat you've left out.

Leaner Cathy wrote in to tell me: *We really enjoy family pizza dinners and have found vegan cheese products very tasty. Even my son says he can't tell the difference in my before and after pizzas.*

My half-sister, Kathy, says this about leaving animal products off her plate:

I went into adulthood thinking I was a healthy eater. I ate chicken (but not fried), turkey burgers, kosher hot dogs, and lots of yogurt and cheese. I drank 2 percent or skim milk, but I never got to the point of being as thin as I thought I should be. In college I studied exercise and physiology, and worked in gyms. But I guess the college drinking and late-night omelets at Denny's outweighed the exercise that I was doing during the day. My weight would fluctuate, but I never looked toned. I was never able to get rid of those last 10 or 20 pounds to look the way I wanted. No matter how much I tried, I was always overweight. I still weighed around 140. This may not sound like a lot for someone who is five four, but it was too much for me.

I went on to get married and have children. My weight sky-rocketed to 170. I went on a traditional Weight Watchers–type diet and lost about 30 pounds. And then I plateaued. I hovered between 140 and 145 pounds and I was wearing a size 8 to 10. Which was okay, but not where I wanted to be.

I tried to eat as many fruits and vegetables as I could and thought I was being "good" when I ate an egg-white omelet. When ordering meals, I would eat the chicken and veggies and not the potatoes and rice. Yet nothing would get me below 140 pounds. I also stopped eating any kind of red meat and thought I was a vegetarian.

Then, when I met my half-sister [author's note: that would be me] in 2004, I noticed how she didn't even eat chicken. She told me about how they had their beaks chopped off and were stuck in pens so cramped together that they could not move their wings. After that, whenever I ate a piece of chicken Parmesan I would have a little picture in my head of the poor beakless chicken.

It was then that things started to click. What resonated most with me was the time my sister and I spent together. . . . I saw the absolute joy and vitality she had with her diet. So I leaned in a little more and I gave up dairy. That was the hardest.

I've been completely vegan for about a year now and I am proud to say that my weight is down to 115 pounds. I am wearing a size 2, and almost every day someone walks up to me and asks me how I lost all of that weight. Frankly, I never saw myself as heavy, but the looks on people's faces don't lie.

People also notice that my skin is much more youthful-looking now. If they ask what I eat I say everything, just nothing from an animal. I eat guacamole and black beans with salsa and a corn tortilla when I go to a Mexican restaurant. I have pasta primavera—no cheese or butter—when I eat Italian. Or eggplant parmesan without the Parmesan (or with a nondairy alternative).

I try not to be a junk food vegan because that's easy to do when you have kids. Speaking of which—I use meat substitutes whenever I can in their meals. They actually say they like the veggie chik'n nuggets better than chicken nuggets.

For dinner I usually make pasta dishes with traditional marinara sauce and use meatless meatballs or mushrooms and veggies. Sometimes we have taco night and I use meatless crumbles for the beef and veggie shreds for the cheese. They are delicious and the kids can't even tell they aren't eating anything animal.

Initially it was really weird for me to think that I could actually authentically become vegan. But now that I have leaned completely in, I would have it no other way. I am hooked on the health aspect and the anti-aging effect that all this has had on my body. I also hardly ever get sick since giving up animal products.

One more thing: I find it really empowering to go to any restaurant I want to and order in a way that is healthy, delicious, and animal-free. My new body keeps me motivated as well.

Extra Lean: Instead of serving up just one veggie on your dinner plate tonight, put three on the plate; you could try butternut squash, kale, and asparagus, for instance, or some other colorful combination! With more variety, you'll likely eat more veggies, and with all that high fiber and water content filling you up, you're on your way to more weight loss.

Extra Lean: Keep a list of local restaurants that you know have food that will satisfy your needs. Then when you are making plans to go out, refer to your "go-to" list.

Bon appétit, my friend!

So, what are you going to do today?

✓ Drink lots of water.
✓ Eat a hearty breakfast.
✓ Eat an apple.
✓ Just for today, say no to your poison.
✓ Go a little nuts.
✓ Trade up the milk and butter.
✓ Put a little flax on it.
✓ Do a deep dive for five.
✓ Switch up your drinks.
✓ Make lunch without animal products.
✓ Take your vites.
✓ Add in some exercise.
✓ Change up your cheese.
✓ Eat a superfood.
✓ Love yourself a little.
✓ Toss up a big bowl of salad.
✓ Make some cashew cream (if it's creaminess you need).
✓ Take the animals off your dinner plate.

Day 19.

Have a Little Fun

TODAY MIGHT BE THE MOST JOYOUS TWEAK OF ALL—AND FOR SOME OF you the most difficult, at least at first. Your prescription for today is to have fun. That's it. Just have some fun.

I'll bet I could tell some of you that you have to drink a potion made with a hundred different herbs that taste terrible and are hard to come by, and that you have to do two hours of hard-core exercise followed by days of fasting and nights in sweat lodges, and you'd dutifully go along with the program. But the suggestion that you have some plain old fun might leave you hard-pressed. And yet today, having fun—*not* herbs and fasting—is exactly the prescription.

Today, I want you to have at least 30 minutes (yes, 30!) of pure, unadulterated fun. I want you to laugh out loud and feel light inside; I want you to be downright playful and silly.

Let me be clear: I know how busy you are, and I know how much needs to be taken care of. I respect that you are beholden to keep your life running well, and that your time is precious. I get it: life is demanding, and you're on a schedule. And yet . . . I want you to set aside everything else and just give yourself a little vacation from your work and chores and "shoulds" . . . It's only for 30 minutes, after all. Today and for the rest of the next 30 days and beyond, you are not only allowed to have fun, you are *supposed* to have fun. (You may not be able to do 30 every day, and sometimes you might be able to give yourself more, but for today, give yourself a solid 30.) Even the Dalai Lama says that the purpose of our lives is to be happy!

Many of us have these funny ideas about what will make us happy. Maybe you think you will only be happy if you lose some weight and become lean. That kind of elusive goal keeps us forever feeling wanting—and wanting things to be different. But what if I told you that it's actually the other way around, that getting a little happiness in your life *first* can help you to lose the weight? Well, it's true. When we are happy, we feel more energetic, we have a zip in our step. This sense of levity often leads directly to a more active lifestyle, which burns more calories, which then leads to weight loss.

And it's not only a matter of burning calories. Feeling good and having fun tends to crowd out time we'd otherwise spend standing at the fridge and noshing, or visiting our favorite fast-food joint. And that's what the Lean is all about: finding ways to crowd out bad habits by filling ourselves up with good ones.

It's true. Getting happy can help us get thin.

Happiness, and lack thereof, is intimately connected with how we eat. Just think of it: When you are depressed, what do you do? You likely overeat unhealthy foods, comfort foods laden with fat and sugar to give you a momentary lift or escape from your feelings. You go for chips and cheese, or cookies and cakes. You go for anything that's going to dazzle your taste buds and take your mind off the doldrums. And of course pigging out on the wrong foods just feeds a vicious self-destructive cycle; it may help lift your spirits for a few minutes, but after a few of these unhealthy binges, you put on weight and become more frustrated and depressed with yourself.

An interesting study was published in the journal *Clinical Psychology* in March of 2008 that demonstrated a strong correlation between obesity and depression; it showed that people suffering from depression have changes in their hormones that could contribute to

obesity. The researchers found that depressed people, with their decreased levels of the hormone serotonin—the feel-good brain chemical—tend to eat fatty and/or sugary foods in an attempt to
self-medicate and restore their serotonin levels to normal. And then,
of course, their poor self-image and lack of self-esteem also make it
more difficult to exercise and eat right.

Happiness, on the other hand, keeps
us away from the cookie jar.

> **Happiness keeps us away from the cookie jar.**

So one of the missing pieces to the
weight loss puzzle, it seems, is to boost
your emotional state, to have a little joy
crowd out the doldrums. When you do something fun, you feel lifted
and tend to take more actions in the direction of your goals. You lean
in ever more closely to being the person you want to be.

I asked my friend, Joe Robinson, author of *Don't Miss Your Life*
and a work-life expert (he coaches people on how to create balance
between work and fun), what he thinks about the connection between
weight loss and having fun, and he said: "Fun and recreation create
life satisfaction and happiness. This could play a big role in weight
loss. People who do a half hour of fun every day are building up positive experiences that offset the negative mind-set that leads to
overeating." He says that we need to have very specific skills and a
plan to avoid the default to rote pleasures (standing at the fridge or
eating in front of the telly, for instance). When we have real pleasures and gratifications, the things that allow us to learn, grow, and
challenge ourselves, we crowd out the bad habits of flipping on mind-
less TV or eating junk food. Reaching for engagement, instead of
food, is exactly what our brain neurons want. Here are a few of the
leisure skills he says are critical to have.

The Six Leisure Skills You Can't Live Without

1. **Intrinsic motivation**. Pursuing and enjoying experiences
   for the pure fun of it, off the clock, takes a different moti-

vation than does the work reflex of external results: you need intrinsic motivation. You do it for the inherent interest, fun, learning, or challenge. Research shows we enjoy what we do and stick with it when the goal is intrinsic. Expect no payoff, and you get a big one: internal gratification.

2. **Initiating.** Instead of being told what to do or watching others doing the living, we have to break out of spectator mode and self-determine our lives to feel gratified. We need to research and plan activities, seek out and try new things, invite others to get out and participate, and if they don't reciprocate, go alone.

3. **Risk taking.** The real risk is not risking. Security is a red flag for the brain, which is built to seek out novelty and challenge. Make the risk intrinsic (meaning the result doesn't matter), and you're able to venture much more because, instead of having anything on the line, you're just exploring.

4. **Pursuit of competence.** Since competence is a core need, it's a handy thing to build and sublime to feel. The idea here is that you want to get better at something—not to show off, not for anyone else, but for your own gratification. Pursuing competence leads you to build your skills at an activity to the point where it can become a passion. It's a fabulous self- and life-sustaining skill.

5. **Attention directing and absorption.** The work mind wants to get everything over with ASAP. The key to optimal experiences is being 100 percent engaged in what you're doing now. That means losing the electronic devices and distractions and putting all your concentration on the activity at hand. The more absorbed you are, the more your thoughts and deeds are the same, and the happier you are. It's called harmony.

6. **Going for the experience.** Observation and hanging back don't satisfy the engagement mandate of your brain neurons. To activate a fulfilling life, we have to participate

in the 40 percent of our potential happiness—60 percent is inherited or due to circumstance—that we can actually do something about: intentional activities. That's the realm of experience. Experiences make us happier than material things because they can't be compared with anyone else's experience. They are personal events that engage our self-determination needs.

In sum, my friend Joe is telling us that when we totally engage in some sort of fun activity—like sailing or painting or salsa dancing— we get absorbed in getting more skillful. And the payoff is that we *do* become more skillful and better at the sport or dance, all the while having a blast. We satisfy a core need to push ourselves by engaging in a fun activity. Note to couch potatoes: watching a reality show is *not* included in the fun activity category! You actually need to get up, move, and engage!

Note to couch potatoes: watching a reality show is *not* included in the fun activity category! You actually need to get up, move, and engage!

Fun activities—dancing, playing volleyball, drawing, or singing in a choir, for instance—bring levity to your life. They loosen up your energy and bring in optimism. But they do more than that; leisure activities help engage you with your own life, thus motivating your weight loss from the inside out, which is always a better bet than feeling forced by outside pressure.

Listen to how my friend Lisa was forever changed when she took up a sport and fell in love with it:

I started training for my first half marathon. It was slow at first and it wasn't pain free, but I did it and I experienced a high like I had never felt before.

I was hooked. The thing was, I didn't want to only run. I wanted to mix it up a bit—try something exciting and new. Since I had been a swimmer the last few years in high school, I decided to do triathlons, and it was the best decision I've made in my adult life! I joined a tri club in the fall of 2009, and did my first sprint race in November of that same year. This sport gave me focus—gave me a chance to get out on the road or in the water and be in the moment. Anyone who cycles knows you can't be on your bike climbing a mountain or riding in traffic and think about work stress.

Plus, there was an additional benefit—the icing on the cake: Not only did I see a major reduction in my stress level, but the weight started to come off! I built more muscle and got stronger and completely reshaped my body.

Don't get me wrong—I've not lost my taste for Oreos or Mexican food. After a hard race, Mexican food is usually my go-to celebration dinner. But now I crave the healthy stuff, and what's more, I pop out of bed at 4:30 or 5 A.M. every day to train with my buddies. I am either in the pool or on a run or climbing one of the beautiful mountainsides near my home and loving every second. I have more energy than ever and frankly more energy than most 20-year-olds I know.

Nothing—and I mean nothing—feels as good as chicking [passing] a guy up a mountain.

So give yourself at least 30 minutes of being fully engaged in a leisure activity today. You can work up to an hour, but do at least half that for now. Don't just sit back and observe, but jump in full force and *play*. In whatever you do for fun, feel the weight of all your responsibilities slip away.

By taking your fun seriously, you will regain a sense of aliveness in your life. You'll reprogram what it means to enjoy yourself, replacing food with activity. You'll create more of a momentum of positive experience.

Here are some more ideas if you are having trouble thinking of what to do:

- Painting, drawing, or art lessons; arts and crafts of any kind
- Kickboxing, martial arts, croquet, bowling, or any fun sport
- Dance lessons or attending a dance group
- Windsurfing, scuba, snorkeling, swimming
- Bird-watching
- Kayaking, canoeing
- Rock climbing
- Cooking class (if it's vegan and healthy!)
- Poker, chess
- Learning to play a musical instrument
- Digging for fossils or collecting certain flowers or rocks
- Making and flying kites
- Taking an acting class
- Gardening
- Needlework, quilting, knitting, sewing
- Billiards
- Ceramics, pottery
- Playing board games with your kids
- Flower arranging
- Golf
- Karaoke
- Writing poetry
- Joining a drum circle

I've recently discovered Wii dancing, which is a video game you can follow along to and then score yourself as to how well your dancing keeps up with the figure on the screen. Not only is it fun to do (with friends even better), but it's great exercise!

On the days you don't do your more formal leisure activity, get out and throw a ball or Frisbee with your dog, or blast some music and dance in your bedroom or sing along while driving. (Rule: you must smile wildly for the 30!)

All these activities send a signal (to those around you, but more importantly, to your own unconscious) that you are opening up rather than closing down. They are guaranteed to assist you as you continue to shift your health habits. Every time a smile breaks across your face, the entire energy of your body lifts.

All these activities send a signal (to those around you, but more importantly, to your own unconscious) that you are opening up rather than closing down.

> ***Extra Lean:*** Take a group walk with friends, or better yet, walk your neighbor's dog who doesn't get out enough and watch that tail wag. Take up biking instead of driving; you'll save money on gas, the environment will thank you, and you'll get some good exercise. Besides, seeing the world from a bike is so much more refreshing than from inside a car.

You don't have to force yourself to be positive; just do things that will authentically make you happy. Mixing up the day with a few minutes of joy here and there will keep you from getting bored or overwhelmed, two states of being that often send us straight to the pantry.

Doing something fun is an intrinsic part of the balance that the Lean is all about. The better you feel physically, the more fun you will want to have; having more fun, you will naturally be inclined to look for ways to share your joy. You will experience a broader view of yourself and the world around you. And you will most assuredly move away from looking to food as a sole source of joy once you experience magnificent multidimensional wellness. You will become more attuned to all the wonder and grace at work in the world and in your life today, and you will find yourself resonating more with that extraordinary energy of lightness. So today, laugh, dance, and do something fun!

So, what are you going to do today?

✓ Drink lots of water.
✓ Eat a hearty breakfast.
✓ Eat an apple.
✓ Just for today, say no to your poison.
✓ Go a little nuts.
✓ Trade up the milk and butter.
✓ Put a little flax on it.
✓ Do a deep dive for five.
✓ Switch up your drinks.
✓ Make lunch without animal products.
✓ Take your vites.
✓ Add in some exercise.
✓ Change up your cheese.
✓ Eat a superfood.
✓ Love yourself a little.
✓ Toss up a big bowl of salad.
✓ Opt for cashew cream (if it's creaminess you need).
✓ Take the animals off your dinner plate.
✓ Have a little fun!

DAY 20.

Pump It Up

I HOPE BY TODAY YOU ARE FEELING A LITTLE STRONGER, AND FEELING more confident that the Lean is actually working. And it *is* working, I promise. With every day, you are making the shifts that are getting your body clean and energized; with every day you are letting go of a little something that used to drag you down.

Because you are most likely feeling fiercer than you have in a while, I thought it would be time to add in some strength. You are burning calories, cleaning out, and nourishing every cell and fiber of your being. Now let's pump up your bod a little. You are going to feel so good. I want you to see what you're capable of today. I want you to start or bump up some strength training.

> With every day, you are making the shifts that are getting your body clean and energized; with every day you are letting go of a little something that used to drag you down.

What Is Strength Training?

While aerobic (cardio) exercise is the most effective form of physical activity in terms of overall weight loss, strength-training exercise is better at toning, defining, and creating new muscle. That's because strength training (also called *resistance* or *weight* training) is all about the process of converting fat, which isn't a very dense bodily tissue (meaning it's larger, and takes up more space on the body) into lean muscle mass, a denser and firmer type of tissue. In a side-by-side visual comparison, a pound of fat is much larger than an equivalent pound of muscle. Converting body fat into muscle isn't just about appearances, though; strength exercises also enhance metabolism, decrease stress levels, increase mental clarity, *and* boost your stamina.

Strength training is a broad term that typically includes any kind of exercise in which you use resistance (weights, bands, even your own body weight) to perform controlled repetitions of specific movements. And to clear up a misconception, strength or weight training is *not* synonymous with bodybuilding. Professional bodybuilders choose to push their strength training to an extreme level, which in highly unusual (yet memorable) cases results in bulky, overdeveloped musculature—not what I have planned for you.

Massive muscle overdevelopment isn't a concern for most people, and especially not for women. Because of the hormonal differences between women and men (women naturally produce less testosterone than men) it's impossible for a woman's muscles to *naturally* develop to the same extent as a man's. Even most men would find it difficult to bulk up their muscles to the degree that some extreme bodybuilders do; the image you may have of excessively muscular men and women flexing and contorting for the camera is almost always the result of anabolic steroid use, not simply using weights or resistance, so don't let fears of "bulking up" stop you from starting a strength-training program.

Beginning a strength-training program may be overwhelming at first, because for many people it's a whole new experience with new terminology, new equipment, or maybe even a new environment; but a little background knowledge will show you how simple it really is to get started.

Getting Started: Frequency and Progressive Goals

Getting tangible results from a strength-training regimen doesn't require a huge time investment; just a couple of 20- to 30-minute workouts per week will give you sufficient results. As with any exercise program, the more work you put in, the greater the reward. Three or more workout sessions per week will yield quicker and more impressive muscle-building results.

In the beginning it's best to start slow and increase your weekly sessions as you become more familiar with how your body responds to using weights or resistance, always ensuring that you allow adequate rest and recovery periods in between workouts. Rest and recovery time varies according to the individual, but as a general rule resting major muscle groups for 24 to 48 hours before working them again is advisable.

If you can only lift a few pounds or do just a few reps, don't despair. The most important thing to remember as you start out is this: strength training too often, using weights that are too heavy, or not taking the time to learn the proper form for the exercises that you wish to do will all dramatically increase your chances of injury. Going to the gym once and using the heaviest weights you're capable of lifting won't magically define your muscles overnight. Building muscle is a gradual, progressive activity. (Kind of fits in with the Lean philosophy, don't you think?) However, time invested in consistent, smart strength training becomes apparent in as little as two weeks. Just think, if you incorporate today's tweak into your program, you'll already be looking more defined by next month!

If you choose to join a gym—which is by no means necessary, as there are hundreds of exercises requiring little or

Time invested in consistent, smart strength training becomes apparent in as little as two weeks. Just think, if you incorporate today's tweak into your program, you'll already be looking more defined by next month!

no equipment that can be performed at home—ask for an equipment orientation, or inquire about free or low-cost introductory personal-trainer sessions. Almost all professional gym facilities offer these services for beginners—they don't want you getting hurt either! Take notes, pay attention to the trainer's advice (especially with regard to form), and don't hesitate to ask for help with a specific machine or exercise if you're unsure how to do it correctly.

Weight Loss and Strength Training

The weight loss benefits realized from strength training lie largely in its effect on your body composition and in turn, your metabolic rate, rather than the actual calories expended while doing it. Cardiovascular exercise is still the most effective way to burn calories. In fact, researchers at Duke University found that participants performing aerobic exercise burned 67 percent more calories than those who did only strength training. This doesn't mean that strength training doesn't increase your calorie expenditure and speed up weight loss; it just means that endurance exercise does it in a quicker and more efficient manner.

So how does strength training help with weight loss? For starters, if done consistently and correctly in conjunction with a balanced diet, some body fat is reduced, and some body fat is converted to muscle. Lean muscle mass requires more calories to maintain than fat does, meaning muscle tissue burns more calories than fat tissue. However, while it's true that "muscle burns more calories than fat" the increase isn't as substantial as was once reported.

The daily metabolic rate for a pound of fat is 2 calories per day, while for muscle it's 6 calories per day. For the average person, this means that 10 pounds of muscle could burn up to 50 calories a day, while the equivalent amount of fat would burn only 20. So while weight training does give you a boost in terms of calorie expenditure, it isn't as significant as diet or aerobic exercise.

Even taking this into account, strength training is superior to aerobic exercise at building and retaining muscle. There are two ways that strength training aids weight loss: it ensures that you retain muscle mass as you lose weight, and it helps to prevent or reverse the natural loss of muscle mass that occurs with the aging process.

This is because your body loses weight indiscriminately; if not prevented from doing so, it will lose both fat *and* muscle. Despite your current or past level of physical fitness, you already have some muscle, and this is the tissue you want to retain. While diet and aerobic exercise are more efficient at helping you lose weight, strength training will help you lose the *right* weight—the fat—while retaining and increasing your body's lean muscle mass. This effect is critical for weight loss; over time, losing muscle instead of fat lowers the body's metabolic rate.

> **Strength training will help you lose the *right* weight— the fat—while retaining and increasing your body's lean muscle mass.**

The body changes as we age, and loss of muscle mass (including cardiac muscle) and coordination, a process known as sarcopenia, begins to accelerate in your 40s. What this gradual loss of muscle mass means is that weight loss may be more difficult as you age, unless you're actively doing something to retain muscle; sarcopenia is by no means an inevitable process. Resistance training is the most powerful way to halt the physical effects of aging. And it's never too late to start: researchers at the University of New Mexico found that beginning a strength training program in middle age reduced sarcopenia's physical effects (sagging skin and muscles, loss of coordination) later on in life and even *reversed* it in elderly people. A separate USDA-funded study found that seniors who followed a resistance-training program for 12 weeks (three 45-minute sessions per week) increased muscle strength an average of 30 percent.

Types of Muscle-Strengthening Exercises

Any kind of exercise in which you lift weights or use resistance to develop muscle is a strength-training exercise. There are four broad categories:

- Body weight (for example, exercise balls often use body weight as resistance)
- Resistance tubes or bands
- Free weights, like dumbbells
- Weight machines (sometimes referred to as circuit training)

It's really a matter of personal preference as to which method you use, but designing a strength-training program that incorporates a variety of exercises from each category will ensure that you're building up more strength by engaging a range of muscles. What's most important about the exercises you choose is that you're maintaining proper form while doing them. This not only maximizes benefits, but is also essential in preventing injury.

Form just refers to doing the exercise correctly, so that you target the muscle groups you intend to work in an efficient and controlled manner. Form is best learned visually, and there are many resources on the Internet that will help you determine how to perform specific exercises correctly, such as the ACE (American Council on Exercise) fitness library at *http://www.acefitness.org/exercise library/default.aspx*, which has videos, descriptions, and pictures. Again, if you join a gym, ask for an orientation to get you pointed in the right direction.

If money is a factor, it shouldn't prevent you from beginning a strength-training program; many body-weight exercises can be done with no equipment, or inexpensive equipment like dumbbells and exercise balls that can be purchased at any sporting goods store or large retailer like Target for less than $20. No gym membership required!

What Is a "Rep" and How Many Should I Do?

Individual weight-training movements are counted in reps, or repetitions, which is the number of times you perform a specific movement. For example, if you're starting out, you might do 10 reps of crunches, which simply means you've done 10 crunches.

A group of reps is called a set. So if you want to do 20 crunches, you might break this down into 2 sets of 10 reps each. The reason that reps are broken down into sets is to allow the particular muscle you're working a slight breather. Weight training is anaerobic exercise (meaning it doesn't depend on blood oxygen levels, as cardio or aerobic exercise does) and it causes lactic acid to accumulate in the muscle, resulting in a feeling of muscle fatigue. Taking a rest between sets simply allows your muscles to clear the lactic acid, lessening the feeling of fatigue.

Depending on how intensely the muscle is worked, the rest period in between each set should be:

- **Lighter weights:** between 30 seconds and 1 minute
- **Heavier weights:** between 2 and 5 minutes

The number of reps you can do depends on your current fitness level and your overall goal. The American College of Sports Medicine offers the following recommendations:

- **Fat loss:** 1–3 sets of 10–12 reps each at an amount of weight that only allows you to complete the desired number of reps.
- **Health and endurance:** 1–3 sets of 12–16 reps each at an amount of weight that only allows you to complete the desired number of reps.

The amount of weight you use will determine how many reps and sets you can do. The idea behind this is called "working to fatigue." The more weight you use, the quicker your muscles become fatigued, and the fewer reps you're capable of doing. Muscle fatigue in this context means that you've worked the muscle enough that you can no longer do the exercise correctly. If you're using the right amount of weight, the exercise will begin to be difficult after about 8 reps, but you'll still be capable of doing a few more. If an exercise is too difficult to even complete 8 reps, you're probably using too much weight.

It pays to design a personalized strength-training program *before* heading off to the gym or beginning a session at home. Planning will not only help you target all the muscle groups that you want to target but will keep you on track by allowing you to set goals and measure your progress. Strength training or any exercise program is more satisfying and easier to stick to if you chart your improvement; consider tracking how many reps, at what weight, and how often you do an exercise to use for comparison as you gradually advance.

2 versus 3 Sets?

To begin with, you may only be able to do a single set of a given exercise, but it's highly likely that over time you'll work your way up to 3 sets, and be able to increase the amount of weight you decide to use. It's much smarter and definitely recommended to emphasize gradual progress over brute force when it comes to weight training. Three sets will maximize muscle-building results.

Muscle Soreness

After you work muscles that have previously been dormant, you're likely to be a little sore. This is a normal condition known as DOMS (delayed-onset muscle soreness). The soreness should only last for 24 to 48 hours, and is unlikely to be as pronounced the second time you perform an exercise. But beware of the maxim "no pain no gain": if muscle soreness lasts for more than 48 hours it should alert you that you've worked the muscles too hard and would benefit from using lighter weights or fewer reps the next time. Always avoid injury.

Results

Most people report that they feel the positive results from beginning a weight-training program after just two consistent sessions if they're using a reasonable amount of weight. In addition to increased energy and stamina, many people report that clothing fits better almost immediately. Results can be less consistent when it comes to actually *seeing* the development and definition of new muscle. Beginning body fat level is one variable. The more body fat you have, the longer it may take your enhanced definition to really show, but rest assured that as your overall body fat percentage is reduced, the muscles you've built will be revealed.

Cardio First or Last?

Doing cardio before weight training or afterward is a matter of debate among fitness professionals, but this doesn't mean it has to be for you. Consistency is essential with any form of exercise. If doing cardio first gets you pumped up and ready for weight training, do it first. If, on the other hand, doing cardio first leaves you too fatigued to do weight training, try doing cardio afterward. Alternately, you could do cardio and weight training on completely different days. The important thing is that you choose a program that you can stick with over the long term, whatever the arrangement might be. Experiment with timing until you find what's right for you, and don't be too concerned with strictly adhering to a specific order.

Warming Up, Cooling Down

Warming up before exercise primes the body for activity by elevating blood flow to muscles and tendons, resulting in increased body temperature and an overall looser feeling in the muscles. This serves the dual purpose of preventing injury and mentally preparing you for the activity ahead. A good warm-up is an aerobic activity, perhaps as little as 5 minutes at a brisk walk or light jog.

Cooling down after exercise is a matter of preference, not of necessity. It was originally thought that the body needed a period of time after strenuous exercise to decelerate in order to prevent muscle soreness or ease the heart back down to its normal level; however, there is little evidence that a cooldown period is absolutely necessary. However, if you need a short period of transition after hard exercise, feel free to take the time.

So today, figure out 3 strength-training exercises you can do for your arms (I always include push-ups, since you can do them anywhere, and it feels right to lift your own body weight), and 3 for your lower body. And give me some crunches, too! If this is too much, lean in by doing just one strength-training exercise for your arms and one for your legs. And still give me some crunches!

Resources

American College of Sports Medicine (ACSM): *http://www.acsm.org/*
American Council on Fitness (ACE): *http://www.acefitness.org/ getfit/default.aspx*
Exercise TV videos: *http://www.exercisetv.tv/workout-videos/*
Free fitness podcasts: *http://itunes.apple.com/us/genre/podcasts -health-fitness-nutrition/id1417*
YMCA (affordable, with branches in many communities): *http:// www.ymca.net/health-wb-fitness/*
So, what are you going to do today?

✓ Drink lots of water.
✓ Eat a hearty breakfast.
✓ Eat an apple.
✓ Just for today, say no to your poison.

✓ Go a little nuts.

✓ Trade up the milk and butter.

✓ Put a little flax on it.

✓ Do a deep dive for five.

✓ Switch up your drinks.

✓ Make lunch without animal products.

✓ Take your vites.

✓ Add in some exercise.

✓ Change up your cheese.

✓ Eat a superfood.

✓ Love yourself a little.

✓ Toss up a big bowl of salad.

✓ Opt for cashew cream (if it's creaminess you need).

✓ Take the animals off your dinner plate.

✓ Have a little fun!

✓ Pump it up.

DAY 21.

Connect the Dots about Where Food Comes From

FOR THREE WEEKS WE'VE BEEN LEANING TOWARD WEIGHT LOSS, AND I'VE been telling you that this program is about doing things as easily as possible, but let's face it. When you've been eating a certain way all your life, favorite or familiar foods can be very hard to resist. If you get a whiff of something appetizing, or if everyone around you is diving into an old favorite, it can be really hard to say no.

Willpower is a tricky thing, and we all too often cave. I've been there. When I think about how delicious some of my old favorite foods are—foods like chicken Parmesan or Brie or eggs Benedict— the one thing that truly keeps me on course is the videos I've watched about where eggs, milk, cheese, and chicken come from. So today I'm passing along my very best advice to you, a weight loss tip that will deliver you to a whole new place in terms of your eating habits: watch a video about how those foods get to your plate. You can find a list of suggested ones in the appendix on page 312.

This is not going to be fun, I know. Get out your tissues. Prepare to be mortified. A lot of truly awful things are done to animals in the (dis)service of feeding humans. But also know that this tweak will be a big ally in your weight loss efforts. Awareness—or consciousness— is such a powerful motivator. Even though you already know that eating a plant-based (vegan) diet is helpful for weight loss, after watching these powerful documentaries (most of them are short, so it won't take much time) about animals suffering as they become food, I'm pretty darn sure you will find it easier to stay on your Lean path.

Think about it this way: if willpower alone were enough for everyone to lose weight, we'd have an overweight/obesity rate of 1 to 3 percent (the rate of overweight/obesity that is caused by genetics) rather than 68 percent. We need more than willpower, and the understanding that our choices are good not just for our waistlines but for our souls can powerfully tip the scales in your favor.

To pick up on our central theme, remembering what happens to animals and all the problems associated with industrial meat production can "crowd out" any desire you might have to eat chicken, bacon, hamburger, or cheese.

That's why today, and for the rest of the days of the Lean plan, your action step is to look at where that food you grew up loving comes from. And then to ask yourself: Does this sit right with me?

The power in deciding to grapple with the ethical issues is that your motivation shifts from being self-based to other-based. The famous psychologist Abraham Maslow proposed that our needs exist on a hierarchy from the most basic physiological needs (for sustenance) on up to basic emotional needs (for love and security) and finally to true self-actualization, the top of the hierarchy. You move on from your own basic physiological need for food to a higher plane of self-actualization as you realize that through what you eat on a daily basis you can actually improve the world, allowing you to live your values every time you sit down to eat!

Suddenly, when your diet is powered by compassion and by awareness about the realities of modern food production, the diet requires no willpower at all. When you're aware of what went into bringing you the foods that you crave, you'll find your cravings melting away under the burning heat of your determination, awareness, and compassion. That awareness will keep you solid—and thin.

Kimberly, who wrote to me, says it well:

My secret, if I have one, is to always think about the animals. Secondly, with just a tiny bit of vanity, is the health effect. There are so many things in the world you can't control, but my eating reflects my ethics and I'm proud of myself. I've always stood up for what's right and my choices now reflect what I know is right for the animals, the planet, and the environment. It's not always easy, in the face of many meat eaters here, but I try to remember that it's not all about me.

I live in Salisbury, Maryland, which is the home of Perdue Chicken. This is a part of the country where it's more difficult to eat vegan than it would be if I were closer to certain stores and products. But, because I don't have access to them, it's made me better at eating a lot more whole foods, avoiding the convenience vegan foods. The health aspect of this diet helps me too because I know that by eating this way, I'll be much more likely to avoid a lot of the chronic health problems associated with eating animal foods. I know I'm responsible for my health and what happens to me in the future. If my current self can respect my future self enough to prepare for the future, I know I'll be better off. I don't want to be sick and miserable in my later years and I know that's my responsibility, nobody else's.

That's what today is all about: connecting the dots. If it's chicken you are hankering for, try watching the videos on how chickens are raised; if you are missing eggs, watch videos about egg-laying hens. Same for dairy; you can Google "factory farm dairy production," and do the same for beef, lamb, and other meats and fish. Mostly, though, I'd recommend you use my list of short films on page 312, as it is pretty comprehensive.

Okay, time for a little inspiration! If you read my last book, you might remember Ben and how he lost weight by becoming aware of how meat and cheese were made. That awareness made his new choices easy, and the weight just dropped off (over a hundred pounds, I might add!). Here's a bit more from Ben:

There were cravings in the beginning: I remember driving past a particular Wendy's in my hometown (on more than one occasion) when the thought of secretly zipping through the drive-through window for some chicken nuggets was almost too much to bear. And the seemingly bottomless package of Kraft Singles that always sat in my parents' refrigerator. And the smell of home-cooked scrambled eggs in the morning . . . I digress.

Even the fiercest cravings could only appeal to my stomach or taste buds, but the pressure I encountered from friends and family felt like it was aimed squarely at my heart.

What kind of person can look his own (Jewish!) grandmother in the eye and say, "No, Grandma, I won't be having any of your Thanksgiving turkey this year"? But I found it helpful in those moments to remind myself of why I changed my diet in the first place. That happened on the day I saw a video depicting baby chicks being debeaked, which for the several hundred million hens born into the egg industry each year means having their beaks seared off by a hot, mechanized blade. The industry, which produces 99 percent of all animal products in America, refers to practices like debeaking as "modifications."

As the blade came down on the birds, one after another, their whole bodies winced in pain. The hand of the worker performing this particular modification moved with such ruthless efficiency that it was clear she had performed this procedure many thousands of times per day over a long, long period of time. Similarly appalling procedures are performed on every species of farmed animal (the dehorning of cattle with a glorified bolt cutter, the tail-docking of baby pigs, the toe-clipping of baby turkeys), but this image has never left my mind.

Reliving such memories can be unpleasant, but it also makes it easier to remain rational and resolute in the face of both internal and external challenges. I would do just about anything to put a smile on my grandmother's face, but it was the images of those animals—sweet little chicks or a docile cow—that made

*me say, "no thanks." How could I enjoy eating something when
I couldn't even stand to watch the process of how it ended up on
my plate? Seeing the slaughterhouse videos woke me up, made
me aware (it chilled me to the bone, actually). It became easy
to pass up those old favorites, a relief. It's like I was released from
some crazy addiction finally, and my mood soared while the
pounds kept coming off.*

*Funny how it was a mental/emotional thing that triggered
the change in how I ate. My weight loss became so easy, effortless really. I still watch online clips and undercover videos from
time to time because I want to stay straight, if you will. I want
to keep feeling good about who I am on the inside, and as a result, keep the healthy slim body I finally have.*

I promise you, these videos will likely be the most powerful mo-
tivators you will ever come across.

So, what are you going to do today?

- ✓ Drink lots of water.
- ✓ Eat a hearty breakfast.
- ✓ Eat an apple.
- ✓ Just for today, say no to your poison.
- ✓ Go a little nuts.
- ✓ Trade up the milk and butter.
- ✓ Put a little flax on it.
- ✓ Do a deep dive for five.
- ✓ Switch up your drinks.
- ✓ Make lunch without animal products.
- ✓ Take your vites.
- ✓ Add in some exercise.
- ✓ Change up your cheese.
- ✓ Eat a superfood.
- ✓ Love yourself a little.
- ✓ Toss up a big bowl of love salad.

✓ Opt for cashew cream (if it's creaminess you need).
✓ Take the animals off your dinner plate.
✓ Have a little fun!
✓ Pump it up.
✓ Connect the dots about where food comes from.

DAY 22.

Blend Up a Power Smoothie

YOU'VE BEEN LEANING TOWARD WEIGHT LOSS FOR THREE WEEKS NOW. You're likely experiencing an increase in energy, you're definitely crowding out the bad stuff by now, and maybe even noticing a slight decrease in your pants size.

Yesterday was probably a little rough. Well, today I'm going to go easy on you. I'm going to introduce you to my delish Power Smoothie.

It's one of my favorite ways to get some protein, a superfood, *and* . . . wait for it . . . a veggie! Yep, you heard that right, a veggie. In a smoothie. You'll get all the benefits of eating something green and wholesome, and you'll never even know it's there.

Get out your blender. Add 6 to 8 ounces of ice-cold coconut water or plain water. I like coconut water because it's fat free, super low on sugar (be sure to get one without added sugar, by the way), and it restores your electrolytes better than the sugary, chemical waters you find on your grocer's shelves. And check this out: coconut water is so close in composition to our own blood plasma that it can be used intravenously in an emergency! I'm not talking about the milk, mind you, but rather coconut *water*. You can also use plain old water if you want to skip the coconut and save a little money.

Toss in a few cubes of ice. Add a scoop of protein powder; I like Vega Sport, Life's Basics, Sun Warrior Raw Protein, and Solaray Soytein because they are not sweetened with anything that will spike your blood sugar. You can find generic brands online or made by your favorite health food store. You want to look for pea, hemp, brown rice, and/or soy; steer clear of whey and casein protein, as they are dairy and not part of the Lean plan.

Next, add in a cup or so of fresh or frozen blueberries. If you need a little sweetener, add some stevia or agave. And here's the kicker: toss in five or six frozen broccoli florets. I promise you won't even taste the broccoli (but definitely use frozen, because you'll taste it if it's raw and fresh), and the purple color from the blueberries will mask the green.

Blend until smooth.

Have this delicious smoothie as one of your snacks, preferably right after exercise. Why then? Because if you feed your body protein within thirty minutes of exercising (the sooner the better, actually), especially strength training, you will help along the process of your muscles' recovery and the building of new muscle mass. The better the muscle mass, the better the calorie burn.

A very common mistake people make when they are trying to lose weight is to skip food after a workout, thinking that fat burning will continue at a higher rate because their appetite is depressed. In reality, it's better to ingest some plant protein immediately after exercise, especially if it's a prolonged or high-intensity workout. A lack of protein will result in unbalanced blood sugar levels, and you'll feel the hunger.

Extra Lean: Don't let yourself get hungry; when there is nothing in your belly or intestines, your body releases ghrelin, the hunger gremlin, which sends the message to go out and get food, any food! Well-timed snacks of a few nuts, an apple, or a Power Smoothie should keep you feeling good.

You read all about blueberries on Day 14, when we talked about superfoods; they're loaded with nutrients and obviously they add great taste. But why the broccoli? Because broccoli's a great cleansing food. It's a member of the cruciferous vegetable group; it creates a phytochemical called sulforaphane, which stimulates enzymes in the liver that detoxify carcinogens before they can damage cells. Broccoli is also a great source of potassium (good for your nervous system and brain function, and it promotes muscle growth), iron, calcium and magnesium, and of course, vitamin C (great for the immune system!). Most exciting about the humble broccoli is that it contains something called indole-3-carbinol, a powerful antioxidant that thwarts the growth of breast, prostate, and cervical cancer.

And as for weight loss, broccoli is high in fiber and helps maintain stable blood sugar, which will stave off the hunger beast.

Here, again, your Power Smoothie recipe:

6–8 ounces water or coconut water
    Few cubes of ice
    Scoop of protein powder made from soy, rice, hemp,
      and/or pea
    1 cup blueberries
    5 frozen broccoli florets
    Stevia or agave to taste (only if needed)

Have it after exercise. And if for some reason you aren't exercising today (remember, you're aiming for 30 minutes every day, even if it's to walk the dog), have it as a midmorning or afternoon snack. You'll be packing in the nutrients while sending the pounds packing.

So, what are you going to do today?

✓ Drink lots of water.
✓ Eat a hearty breakfast.
✓ Eat an apple.
✓ Just for today, say no to your poison.

✓ Go a little nuts.

✓ Trade up the milk and butter.

✓ Put a little flax on it.

✓ Do a deep dive for five.

✓ Switch up your drinks.

✓ Make lunch without animal products.

✓ Take your vites.

✓ Add in some exercise.

✓ Change up your cheese.

✓ Eat a superfood.

✓ Love yourself a little.

✓ Toss up a big bowl of salad.

✓ Opt for cashew cream (if it's creaminess you need).

✓ Take the animals off your dinner plate.

✓ Have a little fun!

✓ Pump it up.

✓ Connect the dots about where food comes from.

✓ Blend up a Power Smoothie.

DAY 23.

Back Away from Sugar

OKAY, BELOVED LEANER, WE ARE GOING FARTHER, HONING THE DIET A bit more so you can pick up even more momentum. As of today, it's fruit first. If you want something sweet, grab an apple, cut up a pear, eat a handful of blueberries. And if you want to bake up a dessert, use stevia or agave as a sweetener. Just by opting for these sweeteners rather than sugar or high fructose corn syrup, you will begin to pull away from the sugar crazies and their assault on your energy and metabolism.

There are so many luscious fresh fruits available year-round now, and getting in the habit of grabbing fruit ahead of other sweet treats is one of the best ways to lean.

Now, I'm not going to sugarcoat this (sorry, couldn't help myself). Do not think for a second that I don't understand what it's like to crave sugar; I do. If I could live on sugar alone, I would. There is something about the pleasure of eating a cookie or piece of cake that cannot be equaled. It's pure bliss, that glorious taste sensation, so much so that you just want it to keep going. And going. And going. It's like chasing after a high that you can never quite reach after that first bite.

But of course it's always fleeting, this sugar bliss. After a short time, you crash and need more. Crave more. Would go to any length to get more. You're tired and cranky and unsatisfied unless and until you get more. And thus the sugar madness is in full swing. Before you know it you aren't just downing a few soft drinks (did you know that colas are not just full of sugar but also contain salt, just to make you all the more thirsty for the sweet taste?), but eating up whole bags of cookies and too many pieces of cake. Talk about crowding out in the wrong direction! Gorging on sugary things fills you up so there's no room for nutritious, fiber-filled food to look, sound, or taste appealing.

I get it, I really do. For most of us, a bowl of brown rice or fresh blueberries just doesn't compare.

But all those sweets are just pounds on the hips. Really. I want to get you out of this madness; I want to help you step off this insane, wild ride that sugar has you on. Because it's not just that sugar makes you tired and cranky, and it's not just that you aren't getting any nutrition from sugar (you get none), both of which are serious issues. Along with sugar come other culprits, like fat and refined carbohydrates, not to mention eggs and dairy—none of which are good for the waistline. After all, you're not eating sugar cubes, are you? You are most likely eating cakes or cookies or frozen treats, and the other ingredients in that stuff are trouble.

Sugar, or glucose, on its own is not really a bad thing; it's the body's source of fuel. But we get all the glucose we need from a whole foods diet that includes grains, beans, and fruits. Our digestive system breaks down the food, and the glucose is released into our cells to power our body and brain. That's the way it's supposed to work. We don't need to supplement our diet with more sugar than that which naturally occurs in whole foods.

At this point you might be asking, "But if beans and grains and fruit convert into sugar when they are digested, doesn't that mean they're not good to eat either?" In a word, no. Those whole foods release their sugar very, very slowly because of the fiber in them, and they don't give you a sugar rush. They feed your cells as needed rather than flood them. (Refined flours, like the flour used in white bread and bagels and breakfast pastries, by the way, do release glucose into your bloodstream right away, and as such should be considered equivalent to sugar. But more on that when we talk about the glycemic index, on Day 26.)

Cakes, cookies, ice creams, doughnuts—these are all intensely sugar- or high fructose corn syrup–sweetened foods. And they do you no good.

Sugar and high fructose corn syrup (HFCS) also hide out in an alarming number of everyday foods like ketchups, sauces, many processed foods, and most sodas and juice drinks. These sweeteners are ubiquitous these days, and there's a reason for it. Sugar and HFCS make the foods they are in addictive. They trick your brain to make you want more. And that's good for business.

> **Sugar and high fructose corn syrup (HFCS) also hide out in an alarming number of everyday foods like ketchups, sauces, many processed foods, and most sodas and juice drinks.**

So good, in fact, that Americans are now eating more than 63 pounds of HFCS per person every year (which translates to a whopping 128,000 calories!). Of nonfood. No matter how much you eat, your body will still crave more food because it's not getting any nutrition.

> **Americans are now eating more than 63 pounds of HFCS per person every year (which translates to a whopping 128,000 calories!). Of nonfood. No matter how much you eat, your body will still crave more food because it's not getting any nutrition.**

The craving is not just about the sugar; it's the effect of the combination of sugar and fat. Here's how it works: sugars and fats together have a powerful drug-like effect—far more powerful than just the sugar on its own. The taste and feeling of sugar on your tongue literally sets off the release of opiates in your brain. The opiates elicit the release of dopamine, which is a feel-good chemical. Whatever you were doing to get the dopamine rush becomes something you want to do again and again as you try to re-capture that "good" feeling. So you return to calorie-laden sugary treats over and over again.

As Dr. Neal Barnard puts it, "They're an especially dangerous combination, because the sugar lures you in, and the grease fattens you up." The mild drug-like effects have been demonstrated to keep you coming back for more, just like an addict comes back for more heroin or alcohol or nicotine.

Now, when you try to give up sugar, that's also a little like an addict giving up a drug, and you might well experience some with-drawal symptoms. You might get headaches or experience dizziness, irritability, and fatigue. You might crave it even more than before. This is because your body will take a few days, maybe a week or so, to regain metabolic harmony.

Before we go any further, let me share with you a little secret that's worked for me, a dyed-in-the-wool sugar addict. This might help you through a tough spot.

As you've probably gathered by now, I don't eat sweets regularly, and when I do they are pretty healthy treats, like brown rice with some hot vanilla soy creamer and raisins or a bowl of blueberries with some warm rice milk poured atop it. I'm also a big fan, as you know, of bit-tersweet chocolate; I'll have a couple of squares or truffles sweetened only with agave and I can usually scratch my itch that way.

But sometimes I indulge. Say it's my birthday and I have my favorite cake (albeit a vegan one, but vegan doesn't mean there's no sugar and oil), and then, because it's so good, I have leftover cake the next day—and who can only have one piece when a whole cake is sitting there? Then I'll have cookies all week long (I have a cou-ple of friends who always make cookies and cupcakes for my birth-day!), and before I know it I'm full on in the throes of sugar madness. By now, my stomach is gurgling from the bloat, I'm not liking my old fare quite as much, and I've gotten cranky and fatigued. Try as I may, I have a hard time "just saying no."

A few years ago I discovered a supplement called nopal cactus, which is said to support lower blood sugar function and take sugar cravings away. Now, if I am in the midst of sugar madness, I take some nopal cactus to get me out of it.

Nopal is a prickly pear cactus that grows naturally in Arizona and Mexico, and commercially in California. Nopales are the edible leaves, which you can use in soups and salads, although I prefer just to take it in capsules. In traditional Mexican medicine, nopal is used for treating type 2 diabetes. In India, they use it for whooping cough and asthma. Some researchers think that it might also decrease cholesterol levels and kill viruses in the body.

While it's possible that nopal may normalize blood sugar and boost insulin sensitivity, those properties are still being researched. All I can say is that it's worked well for me. I like the HealthForce Nutritionals brand because theirs is certified organic and they use a particular species of cactus called *Opuntia streptacantha*, which is said to be particularly good for blood sugar balance. Certainly, though, there are other good brands out there. You might try it for a week as you switch from the high glycemic sugars to the lower ones, and see if it helps. Usually, I'm off it within 10 days and I'm back to normal with a healthy, balanced diet. (Until the next birthday, that is!)

But then you'll be free—and amazed at how great that feels to be out of the madness, and you'll see how much easier the pounds will come off.

Unfortunately, no sweetener is without its issues, but either agave or stevia are certainly better choices. Agave is much lower on the glycemic index—which measures the effect of different foods on your blood sugar—than other sweeteners, and stevia doesn't raise your blood sugar at all. I recommend these sweeteners because they make it far easier to pull out of a sugar addiction. Some hardcore health folks might not like agave, saying it's not much better than HFCS, but here again, I'm all about progress, not necessarily perfection.

Unless you are diabetic or prediabetic, you really don't have to be hypervigilant about tracking down and avoiding sugar and HFCS.

Just say no to foods that have the following listed toward the beginning of the ingredients list:

> sugar
> cane sugar
> brown sugar
> honey
> evaporated cane juice
> turbinado sugar (lots of health-conscious folks get fooled by this one)
> organic sugar (ditto)
> maple syrup (I'm not saying it's not otherwise good for you, what with all the phytonutrients and minerals, but we're talking sugar here)
> fructose
> or high fructose corn syrup (or "sweetener")

If there is a smidge of sweetener in a loaf of bread or in some nondairy milk, go ahead and enjoy it. And if the sugar is not among the top five ingredients listed, it's probably okay. We're Leaners, not perfectionists, remember?

Listen, this is not an all-or-nothing deal. I'd love to see you have fruit for a sweet treat—baked, stewed, or chopped and raw—but I know sometimes you're going to want to give yourself a little indulgence. We all love to celebrate with traditional favorite foods, like apple crumble or chocolate pudding, and I would never begrudge you those delicious special occasions. But even on those occasions, see if you can lean in to better options, and as you do the addiction will let go of you.

Have your apple crumble every once in a while, but make the crust with rolled oats and a touch of whole grain flour rather than white flour crust, and if the apples need some extra sweetener, use stevia or agave. There is a wonderful recipe for chocolate pudding in the recipe section at the back of the book, and it's chock-full of protein (tofu) and chocolate (superfood!), and it's got just a bit of agave to sweeten. Same favorites you might have loved over the years, but better, healthier versions.

My point is, if you are going for a sweet treat, opt for the better ones.

Stevia

Stevia is a South American herb that's 10 to 30 times sweeter than sugar. When it's used in the form of an extraction from the plant, it can taste up to 300 times sweeter than sugar, and it has zero calories. It seems not to affect blood sugar, and has been used in South America for diabetes. Stevia has also been cultivated and used in Asia as an alternative sweetener in everything from condiments to candy.

Green, powdered stevia leaf is the least processed, most natural form, but it tastes a little like licorice. You can also buy it in liquid droppers, which makes it easier to mix into drinks (I make fresh lemonade with lemons and stevia).

So, it's natural, in that it's plant derived, but is it safe? According to the Mayo Clinic Women's HealthSource, the FDA recognizes stevia as safe in moderate doses, but they recommend that until more research is done, women who are pregnant or breast-feeding should avoid stevia, and others should limit their intake.

Agave

Most agave sweeteners come from the core of the blue agave plant, which is processed into syrup. Its taste and consistency are similar to honey, but it registers lower on the glycemic index than honey, and much lower than sugar and HFCS. It's a lot sweeter than sugar, so you can use less of it. Again, you'll hear people say that it's no better than HFCS, but the fact is, it doesn't drive your blood sugar up in the same way, so it's a better choice.

You already know my thoughts on artificial sweeteners.

Although this may seem redundant, I'm going to remind you yet again not to have on hand any treats or foods that make you bonkers. Not in the house and not in your office. Don't buy those cakes and cookies or candy or fudge, and don't order them at restaurants. Why tease yourself by having them around? And remember, one bite is never just one bite! If you want a sweet treat, make something at home. I have a few suggestions in the recipe section of the book.

So, what are you going to do today?

✓ Drink lots of water.
✓ Eat a hearty breakfast.
✓ Eat an apple.
✓ Just for today, say no to your poison.
✓ Go a little nuts.
✓ Trade up the milk and butter.
✓ Put a little flax on it.
✓ Do a deep dive for five.
✓ Switch up your drinks.
✓ Make lunch without animal products.
✓ Take your vites.
✓ Add in some exercise.
✓ Change up your cheese.
✓ Eat a superfood.
✓ Love yourself a little.
✓ Toss up a big bowl of salad.
✓ Opt for cashew cream (if it's creaminess you need).
✓ Take the animals off the dinner plate.
✓ Have a little fun!
✓ Pump it up.
✓ Connect the dots about where food comes from.
✓ Blend up a Power Smoothie.
✓ Back away from sugar.

DAY 24.

Start Seeing Your Weight Loss as Real!

YOU'RE JUST ABOUT A WEEK AWAY FROM DAY 30, AND I'M SURE YOU ARE already doing your own reflecting. Sometimes we just can't even imagine that we could be any other way than how we are now. We simply can't wrap our heads around the idea that change could actually happen, that we might actually become the person we want to be. (Natala, whom you met earlier, says that her 200-pound weight loss was like watching paint dry! It was happening, but she couldn't see all those little changes happening daily.) If you've been struggling with your weight forever and failing too often, it's easy to settle into beating yourself up and resigning yourself to a body and mind-set that just feels hopeless.

Today, we are going to shake that up. You are going to change your mind. Literally. You are going to plant the seeds for weight loss on the mental and emotional levels through *guided imagery*. You've probably heard the term, and perhaps you've used visualization techniques before. Guided imagery is simply using your imagination to facilitate a change in your life. And it can be a remarkably powerful tool as you lean toward weight loss.

When you visualize what you want to see happen, you give your brain new images and feelings to refer to, a new framework that your intention can flow through. I always think of guided imagery as sort of like adding a new track to a toy train set: until you lay new track and pull the switch so the train can transfer over to it, the train is stuck going round and round the same track. Similarly, our thoughts are often stuck on a track of negative or self-defeating images. When you add new "tracks" or positive, goal-oriented images, your mind starts creating a new psychological and emotional landscape.

There's no hocus-pocus here; I'm not saying you can think something and it will happen. That would be magical thinking, and it would be facile and naïve to suggest that you could lose weight without substantial effort. No, this is more about setting your intention to be the person you want to become, and then leaning in to choices that will bring that person about.

Simply put: Change starts with the decision to change, the intention to go a new route. This is about shifting your mind and then letting your body follow.

> Change starts with the decision to change, the intention to go a new route. This is about shifting your mind and then letting your body follow.

As you learn to switch up the internal dialogue and images of yourself, the real world actions follow. You start gravitating more toward habits and practices that support the new vision of yourself. You start looking at life with a new eye, a new perspective, and things just start feeling different. When you rejigger the way you perceive, you show up in your life differently.

When I began to visualize myself as being thin and fit, for instance, I would see myself in my mind's eye as someone who was athletic and who loved healthy food. I saw myself with a spring in my step, bounding up hiking trails. I saw myself talking to people about healthy food I'd discovered, and sitting down to share colorful and nutritious meals. I visualized a flat stomach and lean limbs, and I imagined looking in the mirror and liking what I saw. Those visuals replaced the old ideas I had of myself as being sloth-like, ugly, and addicted to desserts. Regular practice of guided imagery reshaped and replaced the images I had of myself so that I began to know what it felt like to be someone who is "healthy, fit, and happy." I played out in my mind's eye what I would look and feel like, how I would eat and exercise, and how my posture would reflect my self-esteem and newly toned body.

After a few weeks of visualizing myself as fit, I was able to bring that fresh image of myself into my everyday life by doing hikes or workouts and making some delicious healthy food. I became excited at the prospect of change, and everything I did reflected that shift in thinking. I just did things that a healthy, fit, and happy person would do. And it wasn't a big challenge or struggle because I had experienced it all in my mind first. Because I had done mental test runs, had already stepped into a leaner body, when I took it out into the world, it already felt natural. I was in my new body, and it felt right.

What we put out into the world starts with how we experience ourselves on the inside. Think of it this way: if you can see yourself as slim and energetic, you will most probably begin to hold yourself in a stronger and more poised posture. And then you will act in ways that a slim and energetic person would act. You will undoubtedly eat better, exercise more willingly, and stick to your commitments so that the image of yourself is supported and substantiated. And then people will begin to see and treat you as that strong and secure person, which will further energize your new way of being.

Guided imagery is a process that simply puts your energy in a useful and positive place, all the while replacing old messages of self-hatred and shame. It's like creating a map for where you want to go, and then giving yourself new cues—new images and information—so that your behaviors can follow suit.

Here's a guided visualization that will point your energy in the right direction. You can read through it to get the gist of it, and then try it on your own with your eyes closed. Or you can grab a buddy or two and do it in a group, having one person read through the script while you (and the others) give yourself over completely to the mental exercise. You can also record it in your own voice so that you have it on hand to listen to whenever you have a few quiet moments. I do this meditation (or something similar) when I'm dropping off to sleep at night, or traveling and have some time on a plane or train.

A note here: the words may sound a little airy to you, but the tone is designed to relax you so that you can slip into a creative shift in your thought patterns. So take off your cynic's hat and just go with it! You can do this exercise as quickly or slowly as you like.

Guided Imagery Exercise for Weight Loss

Relax and get very comfortable. Close your eyes and let yourself be carried by your breath into stillness, into your creative center. Let the chatter of your mind fade away, and put your focus on your breathing. Feel the air as it enters your nose and travels down through your chest and into your belly. Feel your body as it expands on the inhale and then gently contracts on the exhale. As you enter into this realm of creative thinking, sense your body and mind becoming completely present and alert.

Upon breathing in, say to yourself, "I am." When you breathe out, say, "Leaning in to being healthy, fit, and happy." This is your mantra: I am leaning in to being healthy, fit, and happy. Energize the mantra by putting a slight smile on your face. Repeat the sentence at least three times as you relax further and fall in to the rhythm of your breath.

Now expand your awareness, noting that there is something greater at work than just yourself. You might feel it as an evolutionary impulse to grow, or you might perceive it in more spiritual terms; the important part is to know that you are not the only force at work in your life.

Begin to sense light all around you, as if a positive and supportive force has entered your awareness. You may feel this light as a flood of loving kindness permeating your consciousness. Let yourself open and get comfortable with this flow of goodness that encircles you and begins to fill you up. Feel the potential for a profound shift as you allow yourself to be washed through with all things positive and uplifting. Notice how this light that is all around you sparks to life the light that is already within you. Feel it as it opens your heart, releases your tensions, and lifts you to a higher state of mind.

At this moment, state your intention. Articulate your desire to have a substantial breakthrough in your weight. Be specific about what you would like to experience or shift. As if you are clarifying your intention for yourself, state your reasons why you want the weight loss to happen. Notice if you flinch at any of the reasons, and allow yourself to be completely honest about what you want. Being truthful and integral strengthens the momentum of creation. Plant your seeds in a way that is not demanding or needy, but rather in a way that underscores your lean into personal growth and health. Feel a readiness to have things unfold powerfully yet gently.

And now, let's clear the way. Before any great change or shift, there are undoubtedly fears and mental blockages to overcome. This is your opportunity to push forward. At this part of the exercise, you can speak about any trepidation you might feel about losing weight and being your best. Let it be known to any doubtful or negative part of yourself that all is well and the changes you are making are good ones. Feel yourself becoming free. Feel yourself moving into your own personal evolution. All is well.

In your mind's eye, see yourself as happy, feeling free of cravings, full of energy, and delighting in healthy and nutritious food. See yourself shedding weight and becoming strong. Feel what it's like to have breakthrough after breakthrough. Hear yourself thanking people as they tell you how great you look, how you are just glowing. See everyone around you being supportive and joyful, and note that the healthier you have become, the healthier your friends and family are becoming. Feel the excited energy that seems to have enriched your world. Use all your senses—sight, smell, touch, sound—to make the image come alive. Watch how your life changes subtly and gently, at times even radically, all in the best of ways. And notice that it feels as if this was always meant to happen, that this new you was always just beneath the surface, waiting to be pulled forth.

Look around your inner vision, and see who is in the picture and who is not. Take note of your posture, your new demeanor, how your energy has shifted. Notice how well you connect with people and that you handle every challenge with ease and wisdom. Feel the kindness of your heart as it radiates out. Celebrate the body that you are getting comfortable with. Enjoy the success and let yourself ride the wave of this lean toward ever greater contentedness. See flashes of what you have let go and realize how easy it actually was. Feel this new energy settle into every cell of your being. Add as much color, intensity, and sound to your image as you can. And when you feel a click, as if it has gone as far as it needs to, just let it be.

Now feel some gratitude, realizing your struggle with weight has made you more compassionate and empathetic. You know what it feels like to be out of control and ashamed, and now you can send some goodwill whenever you see someone going through something similar. The struggle has deepened and expanded you, so feel the value of having gone through it.

You're done with the inner work—for today, that is! You just did some very profound tinkering with your thinking. You've taught your mind to go to new places, and you are habituating yourself to positive experiences. The outer will follow the inner, so rest assured this exercise will manifest itself in your healthy bod. Whenever you can, refer back—even if just in a flash—to the strength and flow you accessed, and apply it in your moment-to-moment choices.

Doing this sort of guided imagery is not only uplifting, it is also calming and helps reduce stress levels. I want to emphasize the stress connection once again: numerous studies tell us that if you want to lose weight, you must reduce your stress because stress hormones signal your body to store fat. According to the National Institutes of Health, these hormones—cortisol, epinephrine, and norepinephrine—trigger the release of glucose, increase heart rate, and reduce immune system response. When you are stressed you also have difficulty sleeping, which is also a factor in not being able to lose weight. When you are tired and stressed, you have cravings for comfort food, and thus the vicious cycle of overeating and angst about weight is perpetuated. Meditation (the guided imagery you just did is a form of meditation) significantly improves stress regulation and thus aids in the weight loss process. The relaxation will help you make better decisions and take the emotion out of eating.

You have clearly set your course, and leaned in with the full thrust of your creative mind. Now go out and be the fit, radiant, lean person you know is in there!

So, what are you going to do today?

✓ Drink lots of water.
✓ Eat a hearty breakfast.
✓ Eat an apple.
✓ Just for today, say no to your poison.
✓ Go a little nuts.
✓ Trade up the milk and butter.
✓ Put a little flax on it.
✓ Do a deep dive for five.
✓ Switch up your drinks.
✓ Make lunch without animal products.
✓ Take your vites.
✓ Add in some exercise.
✓ Change up your cheese.
✓ Eat a superfood.
✓ Love yourself a little.
✓ Toss up a big bowl of salad.
✓ Opt for cashew cream (if it's creaminess you need).
✓ Take the animals off the dinner plate.
✓ Have a little fun!

✓ Pump it up.
✓ Connect the dots about where food comes from.
✓ Blend up a Power Smoothie.
✓ Back away from sugar.
✓ Visualize your weight loss.

DAY 25.

Juice It!

COCKTAIL ANYONE?

Veggie cocktail, that is.

Today you're going to drink some veggies. You're going to juice. Or blend (if you don't have a juicer). Another day of powerhouse nutrients that will help you shed pounds.

Why not just eat them, you ask? With grapes and apples and other fruit, I suggested eating them whole rather juicing, right? What gives here?

Well, for one thing, you can take in a lot more veggies by drinking them than you can by eating them. If we want to make sure you get at least 6 servings of veggies per day (because you should get that), drinking some of them guarantees you'll reach your target. I know I would find eating that many vegetables difficult to do, but drinking them makes it easy.

You'll see the list of things you'll be ingesting below and realize there is no way you could possibly sit down and nosh on all of them; it would take too much time and you'd get bored before you were through.

I don't know about you, but when I grew up, I ate the same three vegetables day after day, week after week, and year after year. It was green beans, broccoli, and spinach in our house. But to get the full

182

benefit of the plant kingdom, you really want to have a wide variety of fruits and veggies in your diet. It's good to rotate because each particular fruit and veggie has something specific and different to offer. All those colors and textures represent a wonderful spectrum of vitamins and micronutrients that will benefit your health and weight loss. Remember, the more you fill up with good nutritious stuff, the less room you have for the unhealthy old stuff you were eating before.

Also, when you juice, you are using the whole food rather than just a piece of it. You won't be just squeezing out the lemon juice, for instance; you'll be throwing in the entire lemon, getting benefit from the rind as well as the liquid inside. You'll be using not only the leaves of the greens, but the stalks too; and it's from the stalks that you can get even more vitamin C and calcium (strip the tough outer casing of green on broccoli stalks, by the way, as that can cause gas). And lastly, when you juice, you get the raw nutrients in foods; none of them are lost in cooking.

Just a note here: I'm not a fan of juice *fasting*—where you ingest nothing but juice for a period of days—because I think the body needs food (protein and fiber) to function properly and you can't get everything you need from juices alone. Plus, if you are just consuming juice, you won't be getting enough calories, so your body's metabolism will slow way down as a survival mechanism. You don't want a slower metabolism now, do you? So this tweak is not to be taken as a cue to replace food, but rather as an addition to your daily fare. (There may be exceptions to this if one is doing a short-term healing program under a health care provider's supervision.)

The following is what I use in my daily juice. (Chef Todd Lindeberg came up with this combo, and I love it!) Feel free to adjust the ingredients to your taste, adding in a veggie that looks good at the market or taking out something that doesn't sit well with you. Keep in mind also that you don't want to make the juice too sweet lest you fire up your blood sugar (we don't want to get on that wild ride again!). So no more than 2 or 3 carrots (they are naturally pretty sweet), and since beets have a lot of natural sugar, use them only once or twice a week. If you can, buy organic produce. I know it's expensive, so just do what you can.

THE DAILY JUICE

1 bunch kale or collard greens, chard, dandelion
  greens, or spinach
[A note here: spinach has lots of iron in it, but it's not
  very absorbable, so I prefer kale or collards on a
  regular basis, while working in spinach some of the
  time. Don't cut off the stalks or stems; use it all!]
2 or 3 whole carrots
3 stalks broccoli (save the florets as a side dish for
  dinner or put them in your big salad!)
1 inch gingerroot
1 whole apple or pear (not counted as your daily apple,
  by the way!)
1 cucumber
3 stalks celery
½ bunch flat-leaf parsley
½ bunch mint
1 small beet (every 3 or 4 days)
1 whole lemon or lime

Wash all the ingredients thoroughly and pass through a juicer (I use a Breville Dual Disc Juice Processor).

This is enough for two people to enjoy; however, if you can, drink the whole thing yourself (I do). And drink it right away, as it will quickly begin to lose nutrients. If you want to save some for later, put the juice in a glass jar, filled all the way to the top with as little air as possible (the air will oxidize the juice, sapping it of nutrition), and put an airtight lid on it. Store it in the fridge and drink the remainder within 24 hours. You can have this midmorning or in the afternoon, whenever you feel you need a pick-me-up!

Okay, no juicer? Then blend!

My friend Roxie made me a wonderful blended juice a few months ago, and now it's my go-to drink if I'm just too rushed to juice. Here's what you put into your blender (a Vitamix is ideal—it's a super high speed blender, but they are expensive, so again, do your best with what you have).

ROXIE'S SHAKE

8 ounces cold water or coconut water
2 kale leaves
1 leaf each yellow and red Swiss chard (or any other
 leafy green)
1 lemon (peel off)
1 handful blueberries
1 handful blackberries

The result will be thicker than a juice. That's because there is still fiber in a shake, whereas the juicer filters out much of the fiber. Both are excellent, but you ingest more veggies, and therefore more nutrients, when you juice.

And if you really have no time for the muss or just don't have the funds for all the fresh veggies, try a powdered green drink mix. Go to your local health food store or browse online for green powdered drinks; there are so many good brands to try and some of them even come in travel packs, so they are easy to bring to work or when you're on the road. All it takes is a few tablespoons a day; you can whirl it into a smoothie, or shake it up with about 6 or 8 ounces of cold water or coconut water in one of those plastic cups with a lid. I usually have my green juice at around four in the afternoon, and it just cuts the craving for any of the nasties.

Again, a fresh juice is best. Try Roxie's Shake if you want something a little easier. And if those options don't work for you, have a green powdered drink.

And rest assured, drinking your veggies helps you lose weight (and maintain your svelte bod once you get there). The weight loss is twofold: (1) you'll have more robust energy to exercise and move about, and (2) you'll be filling your belly with nonfattening nutritious juice, which crowds out hunger and will keep you from grabbing for snack food that puts on pounds.

Cheers!

So, what are you going to do today?

✓ Drink lots of water.
✓ Eat a hearty breakfast.
✓ Eat an apple.
✓ Just for today, say no to your poison.
✓ Go a little nuts.
✓ Trade up the milk and butter.
✓ Put a little flax on it.
✓ Do a deep dive for five.
✓ Switch up your drinks.
✓ Make lunch without animal products.
✓ Take your vites.
✓ Add in some exercise.
✓ Change up your cheese.
✓ Eat a superfood.
✓ Love yourself a little.
✓ Toss up a big bowl of salad.
✓ Opt for cashew cream (if it's creaminess you need).
✓ Take the animals off the dinner plate.
✓ Have a little fun!
✓ Pump it up.
✓ Connect the dots about where food comes from.
✓ Blend up a Power Smoothie.
✓ Back away from sugar.
✓ Visualize your weight loss.
✓ Juice it!

DAY 26.

Eat Lower on the Glycemic Index

LOOK HOW FAR YOU'VE COME! GIVE YOURSELF A HOOT AND A HOLLER, because really, you are doing some seriously good work, and I'm more than thrilled you're still with me. You've gone a great distance in crowding out unhealthy, fattening foods in favor of healthier, slimming ones. Well done, indeed!

The process of "leaning in" is about gradually refining your habits little by little so that you get used to better ways of eating in a relaxed manner, with no pressure and no drastic changes that might tempt you to give up and go back to old ways. Now today, toward the end of the Lean plan, we are going to refine your choices a bit more, so that you can decide what to eat, knowing the effects each food you consider will have on your body.

Weight loss is most definitely chemistry: certain foods speed up your metabolism while others slow it down; fatty foods clog you up and make you sluggish, while nutrient-dense, fiber-rich foods keep you feeling energetic and light; and habits like staying hydrated and chewing your food well keep the machine of your body working optimally. To take it a step further, choosing foods according to their ranking on the glycemic index will improve your progress in shedding pounds.

Remember, the glycemic index is simply a scale that indicates a food's ability to raise blood glucose (blood sugar) levels within two hours after digestion. The GI scale ranks foods from 0 to 110; foods with a rank of 55 or lower have a low GI; foods ranked from 56 to 69 have a medium GI; and foods that are scored as 70 or higher have a high glycemic index. For weight loss, it's best to choose from the low to medium GI range, and only eat high-GI foods occasionally, in moderation. Low-GI foods cause a gradual change in blood sugar.

Rather than being an ironclad rule, this index helps us balance our diets. Using the GI to help choose foods doesn't mean that you *never* eat foods that are in the high range; it simply means that you should eat high-GI foods only in moderation. And because we are always mixing different things into a meal—you might have something low GI such as a black bean soup and high GI such as white bread toast—the GI of the meal is actually the average of these two, so it would be moderate. If you had a few pieces of white bread toast and just a bit of black bean soup, the meal would be more of a high GI one.

So it's not a matter of eating strictly on the low side, but rather thinking of how the overall meal will sit with your body's chemistry. The more you lean toward low GI, the more energy you will have for longer and the less hunger you will feel.

> **The more you lean toward low GI, the more energy you will have for longer and the less hunger you will feel.**

And eating low on the GI is not only good for weight loss, but because it keeps your blood sugar stable, it will also help keep your mood steady and your emotions at an even keel. And being emotionally steady will help you continue to make better food choices. See how the momentum of health and wellness builds as you lean in?

How Foods Affect Your Blood Sugar

It's simple. The foods we eat cause a blood glucose response in our bodies, and we can use our diet to have better control of how *quick* and how *high* the response is, and this in turn helps control our appetite. High-GI foods provoke a higher, faster response in our blood glucose level. A rapid increase in blood glucose tells the pancreas to increase insulin levels. In the hours after a meal, this increase in insulin then causes a sharp *decrease* in blood glucose levels, and before you know it, your body is telling you that you're tired and hungry again.

Oregon State University's Linus Pauling Institute notes that 15 out of 16 published studies have found that eating low-GI foods "delayed the return of hunger, decreased subsequent food intake, and increased satiety [feeling full] when compared to high-GI foods."

A major component of a whole-foods plant-based diet is complex carbohydrates such as vegetables, fruits, and beans. Carbohydrates, which were once cast in a negative light because of outdated diet theories like Atkins, are in fact a vital, nutritious part of our human diet. But here's a better way of thinking about carbs: you can classify them in two categories, refined and unrefined.

Refined carbohydrates have a bad rap for a good reason: they include heavily processed foods, such as white bread, candy, soda, sugar, and cake. Refined carbohydrates are rapidly broken down into glucose and digest very quickly, provoking a quick, sharp blood sugar rise and insulin response. Refined carbohydrates are most often found in processed foods because during processing most of the nutrients are stripped away and lots of sugar is added. This might make the food more of a taste sensation, but it's bad news for your weight.

Unrefined carbohydrates, such as those you find in a piece of fruit or a serving of black beans, are metabolized slower. What this means is that the resulting rise in blood sugar and, subsequently, insulin is more stable, and is sustained over a longer period of time. Stable blood sugar and insulin help control hunger.

Dr. Neal Barnard explains the principle: "Low-GI foods can help control cravings. Here's why: a high-GI food (for instance, white bread) makes your blood sugar rise quickly. And what goes up must come down, and as your blood sugar falls, cravings tend to kick in. Many people are on a sugar roller coaster, with cravings kicking in every few hours. Low-GI foods help control cravings, because they keep your blood sugar much more stable." Makes sense, doesn't it? The goal is to stay steady.

Foods and Their GI Values

The following list is not meant to be complete, but represents where common foods fall along the glycemic index:

Quick Glycemic Guide

High GI (avoid or eat only occasionally)	Low GI (enjoy)
White or wheat bread	Pumpernickel or rye bread
Most cold cereals	Oats, bran cereals, Grape-Nuts
Watermelon	Most fruits
Pineapple	Sweet potatoes
Baking potatoes	Pasta
Sugar	Rice, barley, couscous
	Beans, peas, lentils
	Most vegetables

Source: pcrm.org.

You can find a complete list of the GI ratings of everyday foods online, but I'd rather you not get too obsessed with being perfect. The idea is to choose as many whole plant-based foods in their original state (i.e., white bread and most commercial wheat breads are pretty processed, and therefore break down quickly in the body, giving you a jolt of sugar in your bloodstream), and opt for things that don't taste too sweet. It's actually quite intuitive: watermelon tastes super sweet, while apples taste less sweet. Opt for the latter if you can.

Now, here's some especially welcome news: pasta, especially whole grain pasta (I like quinoa- or brown rice–based pasta) brings forth less of an insulin response than does fish or chicken. Isn't that just great news? Dr. Barnard explains it this way: "Pasta is a grain, so it is not especially high in calories, and it has no animal fat or cholesterol. People in Asia or Mediterranean regions who eat noodles every day are healthy and thin. When researchers feed pasta to volunteers, they find that it has very little effect on blood sugar. Therefore it has a low glycemic index value. The reason is simple: unlike bread (a high-GI food), which is spongy and light and very quickly digested, each pasta noodle is densely packed. So no matter how much you chew it, it will digest more slowly, and its effect on blood sugar is very gentle.

"What *does* matter is what goes *on* your pasta. Meat, cheese, and greasy toppings are out. Instead, try linguine with artichoke hearts and seared oyster mushrooms. Or a spicy *arrabbiata* sauce. Or fresh basil, chopped Roma tomatoes, minced garlic, and sautéed shiitakes."

Isn't that just great news? Pasta is not verboten!

Now let's talk potatoes.

Potatoes are a wonderful staple to include in your Lean plan. I especially love yams and sweet potatoes because they are more nutritious than regular white potatoes, and I think they taste better and add some nice color to a meal.

The glycemic index scale rates white potatoes as a high glycemic food, one that provokes a sharp blood sugar response, and so should be eaten only in moderation. However, potatoes are rich in vitamin C, vitamin B_6, fiber, iron, potassium, copper, and manganese.

So if it contains all these vital nutrients, what exactly is the problem with the humble potato? Potatoes can be part of your weight loss plan as long as they're *still a whole food and they're eaten in appropriate portions.*

Most of the time, the problem with including potatoes in your diet lies in preparation methods and portion moderation. Potatoes specifically are problematic because we also tend to fry them in oil or add a lot of other unnecessary things to them—butter and oil, bacon, salt, cheese, et cetera.

Basically, extra processing, added junk, and huge portion sizes are what give potatoes a bad name. A good rule to follow if you want to include potatoes in your diet and still lose weight is to not eat more than a fist-size serving, sans oil and fat (this means butter, cheese, and bacon), no more than once a day. A fist-size serving is about half of a potato. In moderation, roasted, boiled, and baked potatoes can be a great-tasting, filling choice for a whole-foods diet. Now, if it's a yam or sweet potato, have a whole one because they are lower on the scale and more nutritious!

Extra Lean: Quit the "Clean Plate Club"! Leave 20 percent of your food on the plate, and think of it as a way to practice moving away from gluttony. You won't feel so stuffed at the end of a meal, and that sense of lightness will leave you feeling guilt-free and energetic.

Other snacks, like corn chips, cookies (even if they are vegan) and cakes, pretzels, and snack bars are often loaded with refined flours, sugar or corn syrup, and oils. It's best to stick with the snacks on the snack list in the back of the book (page 230) in order to avoid confusion. Again, there is no need to be constantly calculating and obsessing over a list of what you can and can't eat, but today's tweak is that you begin considering where your foods fall on the index. Pay attention, and you'll be surprised at how good and clean your energy begins to feel.

So, what are you going to do today?

✓ Drink lots of water.
✓ Eat a hearty breakfast.
✓ Eat an apple.
✓ Just for today, say no to your poison.
✓ Go a little nuts.
✓ Trade up the milk and butter.
✓ Put a little flax on it.

✓ Do a deep dive for five.

✓ Switch up your drinks.

✓ Make lunch without animal products.

✓ Take your vites.

✓ Add in some exercise.

✓ Change up your cheese.

✓ Eat a superfood.

✓ Love yourself a little.

✓ Toss up a big bowl of salad.

✓ Opt for cashew cream (if it's creaminess you need).

✓ Take the animals off the dinner plate.

✓ Have a little fun!

✓ Pump it up.

✓ Connect the dots about where food comes from.

✓ Blend up a Power Smoothie.

✓ Back away from sugar.

✓ Visualize your weight loss.

✓ Juice it!

✓ Eat lower on the glycemic index.

Day 27.

Cut the Oil

Get ready! You're just a few days away from the end of the 30-day Lean, and today I need to coax you away from something you probably really love: oil. I hate to do it, believe me, but I've gotta.

Let's just say this is not my favorite tweak. I love oils, especially olive oil, and I don't like having to tell you to lighten up on them. I'd happily have bread drenched in olive oil every day of the year. That and a glass of wine! But if you are serious about pushing your weight loss forward, it *is* best to cut back on the oil (all kinds, by the way). It's full of calories and fat and not much else.

Again, I'm not asking you to go fat-free here. You are getting plenty of healthy fats in the Lean plan—from delicious seeds and nuts and adding flax to your meals—but that fat is natural. It comes with the foods; it's just as nature intended it to be. You don't need extra. And it's all that extra we're talking about today.

The truth is, oil is everywhere in your food, whether you're dining in a restaurant or snacking on a bag of chips, and there's a reason. Oil makes things taste good and rich, so it sells food. It's in chips and sauces and prepared meals, and it's hiding in salad bars to make those veggies weigh more so you'll pay more.

Here's the thing to remember: we are primitively programmed to gravitate toward fatty things—just like we are programmed to gravitate toward sweet or salty foods—because in ancient days we needed to grab as many concentrated calories as we could because we never knew when food would be available next. You see, it's not your fault that you like fatty things, like cheese or meat or . . . oil.

Of course as you are well aware, our issue is no longer food scarcity; we need not worry about when and how we get that next hit of calories. Our issue is excess weight and all the health problems that come along with it. And consuming too much oil is a major culprit. So, the sad fact is, if you want to lose weight, it's really important to cut way back on oils of all kinds.

I hear you asking, "But what about olive oil?" It's true that olive oil is a heck of a lot healthier than lard or Crisco, but just because it's better than awful doesn't mean it's good in large quantities. It too happens to be loaded with calories and fat. Olive oil (which really is the best of the oils) has roughly 120 calories per tablespoon, which is on par with butter. If you're trying to lose weight, you wouldn't douse your food in lots of butter (I hope!), nor should you pour oil all over everything either.

Here's what's important to know: oil is not a whole food in itself. It's the concentrated extraction of the fat of many, many plants from which the fiber and nutrition have been stripped out and cast aside.

Olive oil is mostly monounsaturated fat—75 percent actually—and that fat is not at all essential for the body, so you get no bang for the buck, no nutrition for the calories. Then there is 11 percent polyunsaturated fat—not bad for you really, but nothing you need, so again it's empty calories. Then there is the rest of it: 14 percent of olive oil is actually saturated fat, the kind we try to avoid as much as we can. Saturated fat clogs the arteries and raises cholesterol; it's one of the things we consider when avoiding meat and chicken. True, there is a tad (1 percent) of omega-3 fat in there, and that *is* good stuff. But you can get much more omega-3 from flax, walnuts, avocados, and algae supplements if you are looking for it, plus you get all that fiber and nutrition at the same time.

I know what you are thinking: *But I need taste!* True that. And let me repeat that I'm not saying give up oil completely; I'm saying cut back as much as you can without feeling deprived. Or angry.

I don't want you to bounce back to your old ways because you feel like you can't enjoy a pasta dish or a veggie stew at a restaurant. I don't want you fretting about the exact amount of oil they use back in the kitchen. You can't live that way, and I don't want you to.

Just make a conscious effort to refrain from drizzling oil all over your food as a habit. Today, say no to the chips and the dips and the sauces and the fried stuff. Just replacing chips with other healthy snacks (I have a bunch of ideas for you in the What to Eat section) alone is going to hugely affect your weight loss. Here's a simple way to think about recognizing oily foods, too: if it looks slick and shiny, it's got a lot of oil on it. If a dish is glistening, say "no thanks."

When you do use oil to cook with, the best choices are extra-virgin olive oil or organic cold-pressed canola oil, used sparingly. When dining out, get your dressing on the side and order things very lightly sautéed. When cooking at home, use just as much as you need in order for your food to taste good.

What to use instead of oil? Try a cooking spray, but use only a quick shot; don't drench the food or the skillet. You can also sauté with vegetable broth, wine, or orange juice.

I think you might be surprised at how good things taste when you start seasoning with chopped or sun-dried tomatoes, fresh garlic, caramelized onions, vinegars, or fresh fruit (I love mango salsa and plantains to season dishes). Cut back on oil and witness the difference on the scale.

You've met Natala; now here's her husband, Matt's story:

While I have been more focused on my overall health rather than my weight, I've lost around 100 pounds by leaning in to healthy eating. More importantly I'm feeling better than ever. I have a consistent sustaining energy throughout the day and I sleep better at night. I no longer have sleep apnea and I no longer suffer from severe acid reflux.

In the past, I had become more and more concerned with my weight but thought losing weight and getting healthy was hopeless. So I did all I could to ignore my health while making tiny but relatively insignificant changes. All the health claims I'd heard seemed to conflict with each other and none of them seemed interesting to me.

But I started to think seriously about changing my diet after my wife experienced a dramatic improvement in her fight against type 2 diabetes. Our life together until that point was one failed medical strategy after another. With each new doctor, her diabetic condition only worsened. A friend introduced her to some books on the health benefits of a plant-based diet and pretty soon she was off insulin. Not long after that, she was off the rest of the medicines for chronic conditions. For the first time in my life I witnessed health advice that actually worked. The more we looked into it together, the more it made sense. We learned how people that consume little or no animal products experience the lowest rates of preventable diseases.

I wasn't sure I wanted to be vegan; the whole idea seemed so impossible to me. But I wanted to get healthier, so I decided to experiment a bit. I learned that red meat was one of the more dangerous things I ate so I decided to see if I could go a week choosing something healthier. After a week or so I missed it, but I knew I didn't need it.

I found out that dairy was really harmful so I tried to find ways to reduce it. I tried a couple of different milk alternatives and liked the taste of rice milk. By just replacing that one ingredient I had seven healthier meals a week. Pretty soon my tastes changed and I didn't even like the flavor of normal milk. It tasted sour and nasty no matter how fresh it was.

Cheese was a lot more difficult to give up. I tried a lot of the vegan cheeses. Some were horrible, but a few of them, if mixed into a meal, tasted close enough to the real thing. Pretty soon I didn't have those strong cravings for dairy cheese anymore.

I kept eating white meat and fish for a while but soon learned that they weren't as healthy as I thought. They contain almost as much cholesterol as red meat. I really liked the idea of getting rid of as much cholesterol as possible so I started making other choices. I tried a lot of the vegan meat alternatives and enjoyed them enough to say goodbye to meat.

The changes I began to see in my body weren't immediate. But after a few weeks I had to start shopping for smaller clothes. When I hit different milestones I was genuinely excited and surprised. I never beat myself up for not losing more or losing weight too slowly. I was just happy that I was feeling more energy than before. I saw the whole thing as an experiment—I didn't really believe that I would eventually lose as much weight as I did!

Over the next several months I was losing weight at a steady pace but pretty soon I hit a plateau. Even with exercise my weight stopped dropping. I learned that by eating highly processed foods and oil I was eating more calories than my body could handle. I started cutting out processed foods and reducing oil in my diet as much as I could. I found that I could eat meals that were much more satisfying, but had far fewer calories. That's when I started dropping weight again and feeling even better.

I used to love big hamburgers, roast beef sandwiches, and pizza. I loved Italian food as long as it was loaded with mozzarella. I loved sushi and pho and Chinese takeout. I ate huge burritos and quesadillas several times a week. Health food for me meant grilled chicken topped with cheese over pasta or a roasted turkey sandwich with one slice of cheese instead of two. I loved fast-food breakfasts, though I gave them up for coffee shop breakfasts, which I thought were healthier.

I didn't stop liking all that food overnight. I wish it had been as easy as that. It took weeks of leaning in to my new way of eating and substituting new foods for old. If I had tried to change my diet overnight it would have been impossible. When I experimented with giving up foods I still craved them, and badly. But over time the cravings got less and less. In a few months, restaurant commercials on TV lost their appeal.

The real secret for me wasn't to replace foods but rather to change what tastes good to me. Now a meal full of my favorite vegetables, rice, and beans tastes absolutely amazing. I would choose a low-fat, low-sodium, no-oil burrito loaded with beans, salsa, and veggies over a salt-and-oil-drenched fast-food burrito any day. Not because I'm denying myself, but because it actually tastes that much better to me.

In the process I definitely had my share of setbacks; I'm not perfect, but I continue to lean forward. Some of my tips for continuing to lean in are to make friends with your kitchen and learn to make a meal for yourself. Don't count on your spouse or significant other to cook for you. Don't expect them to even want to eat what you cook.

Here's my essential shopping list: frozen veggie mixes, frozen brown rice, tortillas, canned beans (salt free if possible), and any sauces that look tasty, usually a hot sauce, barbecue sauce, tomato sauce, and a low-fat salad dressing or two. Beyond that, I usually buy some fresh spinach, mushrooms, and hummus.

Then when I need a quick meal I throw half a bag of frozen veggies into a frying pan with a bit of water (no oil necessary). Once they're hot, I add half a can of beans. Once it's hot, I slowly add whatever sauce I'm in the mood for, tasting it as I go. I serve it over a tortilla or brown rice and sometimes chop up an avocado over it.

I've made that in a dozen different kitchens (I travel all the time). I've made it with a microwave and I've made an endless number of variations with different veggies, beans, sauces, and

grains. I've had a few failed experiments but those are well worth
the cost of improving my health. Besides, with enough hot sauce
almost any dish can be rescued!

So, what are you going to do today?

✓ Drink lots of water.
✓ Eat a hearty breakfast.
✓ Eat an apple.
✓ Just for today, say no to your poison.
✓ Go a little nuts.
✓ Trade up the milk and butter.
✓ Put a little flax on it.
✓ Do a deep dive for five.
✓ Switch up your drinks.
✓ Make lunch without animal products.
✓ Take your vites.
✓ Add in some exercise.
✓ Change up your cheese.
✓ Eat a superfood.
✓ Love yourself a little.
✓ Toss up a big bowl of salad.
✓ Opt for cashew cream (if it's creaminess you need).
✓ Take the animals off the dinner plate.
✓ Have a little fun!
✓ Pump it up.
✓ Connect the dots about where food comes from.
✓ Blend up a Power Smoothie.
✓ Back away from sugar.
✓ Visualize your weight loss.
✓ Juice it!
✓ Eat lower on the glycemic index.
✓ Cut the oil.

DAY 28.

Do Something Purposeful

Just a couple more days! Yahoo!

Today we're going to lean in another way that's not directly about food. All you need to do is "think of the big picture."

Now, I know this may be hard to think about on those days when you look in the mirror and obsess about what you see, about how upsetting it is that you aren't all the way there yet. When what you really want is to look good in a pair of jeans. First things first; I get that. *Let's take care of how my body looks,* we think, *and then I can be a force for change in the world.*

But maybe it doesn't work like that. Maybe getting your mind off food and cravings and aesthetics by doing something that has a little meaning moves you toward your weight loss and health goals. I've certainly found that to be true.

We already know your intention, which is to lose weight and be healthy. You have already undertaken many wonderful steps to get you there. You are fighting against your instinct to berate yourself as it is, so wouldn't it be nice to step away from all that—if only for a small window during the day—and feel as if your life is powerful today?

Because it is and you are. And the more you *feel* how powerful and effective you really are, the less time and energy you'll devote to pondering whether or not to have another cupcake. I find that many people are bored and uninspired with their lives. Life is frustrating, and there's not much we can do about it. So we eat. And the bad food we eat depresses our energy, and the boredom and lack of inspiration continue. A vicious cycle if ever there was one.

Let's do a little thought experiment: Say you have one year to live. You have one year to leave your mark on the world. What would you do? Let's see what shakes out when you answer the following questions:

1. Is there a relationship that you feel needs some closure?
2. Is there someone you want to (lovingly) communicate something important to—a truth that would help you and/or her grow?
3. Is there some suffering that you could help to alleviate in another?
4. Is there an issue that has always gotten under your skin, something you wish you could devote some time to?
5. Is there anything you could do right now that would make the world better and kinder?

If you knew you had a year to live, wouldn't you want to know you used your life well? Because as much as life is about having fun and accomplishing goals and working hard, it's also about contributing to an evolving universe. There's something that just clicks into gear when you do something to benefit the greater good. You feel strong and vigorous. You feel like you're living on purpose.

I know when I'm feeling down on myself the best remedy—far better than the temporary pleasure of the cupcake—is to make myself useful. It feels great to do something that benefits someone else. It gets me out of my head and into action. I lose that self-centered angst and start feeling charged up, realizing that I'm a valuable person in the world who shouldn't just sit on the sidelines and let life play out without my two cents.

Sure enough, when I remember that I'm on this planet for a reason, that life is not just about the silly, superficial things I get caught up in, time slips away, endorphins fire, and I notice that I haven't thought about my obsession (whether it's the sugar frenzy or hating the way I look) for a while.

If I walk a neighbor's pent-up dog, I feel I've been useful. If I write a blog and share some inspiration, I feel empowered. When I help someone in the store with their food choices, I feel like I'm living with a reason and that I'm a positive force in the world. And that inner strength builds my character, takes me away from obsessions and compulsions and bad habits.

I think about the great people who have changed the world for the better, and I realize they had bigger things to do than chow down on a bucket of chicken or a tub of ice cream. Why not lean toward that kind of life?

Answer those questions above for yourself, and see if there is something you can do every day that will keep you feeling on track.

Ask yourself today and every day: What can I do today that makes my life purposeful? And just do one little (or big!) thing that nudges you in the direction of being a positive force. You'll feel something shift. You'll find out what attributes you really do have and realize that there's something bigger going on than your daily complaints. You'll also feel more positive about the changes you are making and more able to maintain the upward thrust of adjustment.

> **Ask yourself today and every day: What can I do today that makes my life purposeful?**

A word here: I am *not* saying that you don't have reason to be frustrated or unhappy. Nor am I proposing that you don't already do great things with your life. I'm just reminding you—just as I need constant reminding—that the more we move away from self-centeredness, the better we're going to fare—with the Lean and with everything else in life. And busy-ness *will* keep your hand out of the cookie jar, too.

So, what are you going to do today?

- ✓ Drink lots of water.
- ✓ Eat a hearty breakfast.
- ✓ Eat an apple.
- ✓ Just for today, say no to your poison.
- ✓ Go a little nuts.
- ✓ Trade up the milk and butter.
- ✓ Put a little flax on it.
- ✓ Do a deep dive for five.
- ✓ Switch up your drinks.
- ✓ Make lunch without animal products.
- ✓ Take your vites.
- ✓ Add in some exercise.
- ✓ Change up your cheese.
- ✓ Eat a superfood.
- ✓ Love yourself a little.
- ✓ Toss up a big bowl of salad.
- ✓ Opt for cashew cream (if it's creaminess you need).
- ✓ Take the animals off the dinner plate.
- ✓ Have a little fun!
- ✓ Pump it up.
- ✓ Connect the dots about where food comes from.
- ✓ Blend up a Power Smoothie.
- ✓ Back away from sugar.
- ✓ Visualize your weight loss.
- ✓ Juice it!
- ✓ Eat lower on the glycemic index.
- ✓ Cut the oil.
- ✓ Do something purposeful.

DAY 29.

Schedule Your Day

NOW THAT YOU'VE BEEN AT THIS FOR FOUR FULL WEEKS, YOU'VE IN-corporated 28 new tricks into your Lean plan. Today it's time to get organized, to put it all together so that you can keep leaning with ease. I find it really helps to have a plan laid out in front of you, something you can refer to throughout the day to be sure you're on track.

I know I've given you a lot to think about, and some of it is bound to get lost in the shuffle if you don't budget your time and remind yourself of what needs to happen. This is kind of fun be-cause you can see how all the pieces of the wellness puzzle are coming together. When you get everything in writing, you'll see that you have quite a holistic plan, which addresses each of the areas of body, mind, and soul. I'm going to show you what my day looks like so you can get a feel for how the Lean plan can flow, but arrange yours *according to your own needs*. Be sure that you sched-ule each of your three square meals because remember, we want to keep you from getting hungry. We want your energy to stay steady and robust so that you never give the hungry beast a chance to rear its head again.

Kathy's Daily Lean Schedule

6:30	Rise and shine! Drink water.
6:35	Quick visualization.
6:45	Drink water (squeeze of lemon or lime).
7:00	Breakfast and coffee or tea. Take vites.
7:45	15-minute brisk walk or hike; 15 minutes of strength training; drink water.
8:15	Power Smoothie.
10:00	Drink water.
11:00	Have some nuts.
11:30	Drink water.
12:00	Big salad.
12:00	Lunch. Add flax to soup. Take vites.
2:30	Have an apple.
2:30	Drink water.
3:30	Drink water.
4:00	Have a superfood (handful of goji berries).
4:30	Love myself a little (3 minutes).
4:30	Have a green juice.
5:00	Drink water.
5:30	Shoot some hoops in the driveway or Frisbee with a friend for something fun.
6:00	Drink water.
6:30	Dinner.
7:00	Brisk walk after dinner; take my neighbor's dog for a walk (doing something purposeful).
7:30	Watch a video; drink water.
9:30	Do a deep dive for 5 minutes.
10:00	Drink water.
10:30	Bedtime!

Fill in the blanks with all your work responsibilities and appointments so that you've budgeted your time effectively. There are times when you won't do everything every day. For instance, I only make cashew cream once in a while, so that might not be on my daily schedule. I only do strength training three times a week. I'm pretty much off sodas, so I don't bother with that. And nondairy cheese is a treat only every so often and would appear on the schedule as part of my grocery shopping. And some days, the fun I have consists of driving home to some favorite music and rocking out despite how silly I look. Sometimes work is crazy, and I just do the best I can. But the important thing is that the basics are always there: I always have my three squares, each of which includes a plant-based protein. I always drink water. Always have an apple or pear. Always a superfood. You get the drift? You do what you can by leaning in to it, and the schedule will help.

I've provided you with seven days' worth of blank day planners; you can cut out the pages from the book and fill the spaces in and carry your plan with you or photocopy them and do the same.

As you plan out the week, you might want to jot down some menu ideas in advance so you aren't caught hungry and off guard. I always know a black bean tostada with salsa is super easy and quick, and I always have soups or chili that I've made and frozen. Start putting your pieces of the puzzle together, and see how your newly designed life starts shaking out!

6:30 a.m.	
7:00	
7:30	
8:00	
8:30	
9:00	
9:30	
10:00	
10:30	
11:00	
11:30	
12:00 p.m.	
12:30	
1:00	
1:30	
2:00	
2:30	
3:00	
3:30	
4:00	
4:30	
5:00	
5:30	
6:00	
6:30	
7:00	
7:30	
8:00	
8:30	
9:00	
9:30	
10:00	
10:30	

6:30 a.m.	
7:00	
7:30	
8:00	
8:30	
9:00	
9:30	
10:00	
10:30	
11:00	
11:30	
12:00 p.m.	
12:30	
1:00	
1:30	
2:00	
2:30	
3:00	
3:30	
4:00	
4:30	
5:00	
5:30	
6:00	
6:30	
7:00	
7:30	
8:00	
8:30	
9:00	
9:30	
10:00	
10:30	

| 6:30 a.m. |
| 7:00 |
| 7:30 |
| 8:00 |
| 8:30 |
| 9:00 |
| 9:30 |
| 10:00 |
| 10:30 |
| 11:00 |
| 11:30 |
| 12:00 p.m. |
| 12:30 |
| 1:00 |
| 1:30 |
| 2:00 |
| 2:30 |
| 3:00 |
| 3:30 |
| 4:00 |
| 4:30 |
| 5:00 |
| 5:30 |
| 6:00 |
| 6:30 |
| 7:00 |
| 7:30 |
| 8:00 |
| 8:30 |
| 9:00 |
| 9:30 |
| 10:00 |
| 10:30 |

6:30 a.m.	
7:00	
7:30	
8:00	
8:30	
9:00	
9:30	
10:00	
10:30	
11:00	
11:30	
12:00 p.m.	
12:30	
1:00	
1:30	
2:00	
2:30	
3:00	
3:30	
4:00	
4:30	
5:00	
5:30	
6:00	
6:30	
7:00	
7:30	
8:00	
8:30	
9:00	
9:30	
10:00	
10:30	

6:30 a.m.	
7:00	
7:30	
8:00	
8:30	
9:00	
9:30	
10:00	
10:30	
11:00	
11:30	
12:00 p.m.	
12:30	
1:00	
1:30	
2:00	
2:30	
3:00	
3:30	
4:00	
4:30	
5:00	
5:30	
6:00	
6:30	
7:00	
7:30	
8:00	
8:30	
9:00	
9:30	
10:00	
10:30	

6:30 a.m.
7:00
7:30
8:00
8:30
9:00
9:30
10:00
10:30
11:00
11:30
12:00 p.m.
12:30
1:00
1:30
2:00
2:30
3:00
3:30
4:00
4:30
5:00
5:30
6:00
6:30
7:00
7:30
8:00
8:30
9:00
9:30
10:00
10:30

6:30 a.m.
7:00
7:30
8:00
8:30
9:00
9:30
10:00
10:30
11:00
11:30
12:00 p.m.
12:30
1:00
1:30
2:00
2:30
3:00
3:30
4:00
4:30
5:00
5:30
6:00
6:30
7:00
7:30
8:00
8:30
9:00
9:30
10:00
10:30

So, what are you going to do today?

✓ Drink lots of water.
✓ Eat a hearty breakfast.
✓ Eat an apple.
✓ Just for today, say no to your poison.
✓ Go a little nuts.
✓ Trade up the milk and butter.
✓ Put a little flax on it.
✓ Do a deep dive for five.
✓ Switch up your drinks.
✓ Make lunch without animal products.
✓ Take your vites.
✓ Add in some exercise.
✓ Change up your cheese.
✓ Eat a superfood.
✓ Love yourself a little.
✓ Toss up a big bowl of salad.
✓ Opt for cashew cream (if it's creaminess you need).
✓ Take the animals off the dinner plate.
✓ Have a little fun!
✓ Pump it up.
✓ Connect the dots about where food comes from.
✓ Blend up a Power Smoothie.
✓ Back away from sugar.
✓ Visualize your weight loss.
✓ Juice it!
✓ Cut the oil.
✓ Eat lower on the glycemic index.
✓ Do something purposeful.
✓ Schedule your day.

Day 30.

Make Progress, and Don't Worry about Perfection

OH, MY FELLOW LEANER, LOOK AT HOW YOU'VE RISEN TO THE CHALLENGE! You've made it to Day 30 and you are still in the game. You've leaned into a new way of eating and thinking, and you've crowded out some old habits with better-informed ones. Bravo, you!

Habits are a funny thing, you know. They are influenced by emotions and have physiological roots, too, as you've discovered throughout this book. You can't just snap your fingers and change something that's as deeply ingrained as what and how you eat. You have to retrain yourself, slowly and with intent. And also with patience.

> **Extra Lean:** Make a plan for what you are going to eat for the week so that you don't suddenly find yourself hungry and foraging for food (dangerous situation, especially if you head for the grocery store!).

You can't just delete a habit—something you've been doing for many, many years—without putting something else in its place; and in these 30 days, you have done just that. You're drinking lots of water, eating three meals a day without animal products, snacking on fruits and nuts; you're exercising and even doing a bit of meditation. Now give yourself time to settle in and find your footing as you continue on this path of weight loss and healing. After all, you are undertaking nothing less than your own personal revolution of body, mind, and soul, and that takes a moment (or a few months or a year) to take root and be reconciled with the rest of your life.

Nothing good comes from forcing things before their time.

I believe in leaning in to change; it's the only way that's ever worked for me. I remember when I first decided I wanted to get fit, and how I knew I had to change the way I was eating. But there was such a big gap between the way I was living and the way I wanted to live. So I just set my sights on it and then leaned in. Gradually, by taking small but interconnected steps over the course of a few years, I lost my old taste cravings while discovering unbelievably delicious new foods.

Had I pushed myself to go whole hog (pardon me), I'm pretty sure I would have been overwhelmed by the huge change and ultimately given up. I know this method will work for you, too.

Extra Lean: Don't beat yourself up for slipups and setbacks. They happen. If you overdo it at dinner one night or just can't resist your mother's feast at the family get-together, just take a beat, breathe, try to understand what happened, and start again tomorrow. Far better to show yourself a little compassion than to use the slipup as an excuse to go back to old ways.

What I know for sure, and what I hope you know, too, is that when something is truly good for your body, it's also good for your

> **When something is truly good for your body, it's also good for your soul. When you eat food that is grown in the ground or on trees, your body thrives.**

> **Weight loss should never come at the cost of your health.**

soul. When you eat food that is grown in the ground or on trees, your body thrives. When you steer clear of the junk that is marketed to you in advertising and in fast-food joints, you feel energetic and clear, and your body finds its perfect weight and size. Weight loss should never come at the cost of your health. Nor should you ever have to compromise what's in your heart just to be thinner.

I know there are challenges. This is not an altogether easy process. At least not all the time. If you cook at home, you will need to make some adjustments in the way you shop and how you pull a menu together.

Extra Lean: If you are making a soup or casserole, make twice what you need and freeze the rest so that you have some ready-made meals for the weeks to come.

For sure you'll save money, both on food and on health care costs you'll suddenly find you no longer have. But for many of you, as it was for me, it will not always be easy to find good, healthy food. You may sometimes be at a loss for what to eat at a party, or if you are traveling, you'll realize that planning ahead is essential.

All this is workable, of course, and well worth the effort. You can bring your own food to family or work functions and share it with everyone, introducing them to veggie burgers or your delicious salad with everything colorful and crunchy in it. You can seek out ethnic restaurants like Thai or Japanese that offer lots of rice, tofu, and veggie dishes, or go for Mexican black beans with salsa on a crisp tortilla, with sliced avocados and rice. You can certainly take out from salad bars, which usually offer grains and beans along with all the other fixings. You can ask your waiter to bring pasta with tomato sauce, a baked potato with veggies, or a plate of white beans or lentils with everything green there's to be had in the kitchen.

Extra Lean: When eating out, ask the waiter to cut the meal in half and put the extra in a to-go container for the next day. Or split the entrée with a friend.

Extra Lean: If you're out at a restaurant, tell your server you have a milk allergy so that she or he will take your request for no dairy seriously. No restaurant wants a full-scale allergic reaction on their hands!

If you're going to a party, eat before you go, so you will neither go hungry if everything is highly caloric and meaty nor be tempted by foods that are bad for you. And try to keep fruit and nuts on hand for those food emergencies.

Trust me, if there is a will, there is a way! It should be easier to eat healthfully, without a doubt, and while it's not yet, society is making strides in the right direction. But you are out in front, and pioneers are always the ones to be resourceful.

The landscape is shifting, and there is definitely change afoot in our society's nutritional awareness and the availability of healthy foods. You'll find small companies popping up all over the place, providing the sort of delicious, fiber-rich, nutrient-dense food that we've talked about in the pages of *The Lean.*

Listen and you'll start to notice more people making requests for "plant-based" or vegan fare, "sugar-free" and low oil. You might notice a lot of this noise is coming from the younger generation, who are not as willing to go along with the status quo and eating what we have grown accustomed to. More and more people are getting informed and smart about the effects of food, and it's happening; we are getting closer to the tipping point where it will be totally easy to eat well.

But of course change is a big process, especially when money is at stake. There are powerful interests working against your progress, groups that are focused on pushing certain kinds of foods—meats, dairy, eggs, and sugar—so that they continue to profit. The USDA, after all, is an organization focused on promoting and marketing agricultural products.

"I had hoped that the USDA would be able to give Americans the clear advice about diet that they deserve," says Dr. Walter Willett, Fredrick John Stare Professor of Epidemiology and Nutrition and chair of the Department of Nutrition at Harvard School of Public Health. "However, the continued failure to highlight the need to cut back on red meat and limit most dairy products suggests that 'Big Beef' and 'Big Dairy' retain their strong influence within this department. Might it be time for the USDA to recuse itself because of conflicts of interest and get out of the business of dietary advice?"

But alas, we don't have time to wait for the monumental changes that would need to occur in the political system before we start changing the way we eat. We are our own best advocates, following an inner compass as to what's right for us.

In this monthlong process, you've moved away from eating poultry, red meat, fish, and eggs, and replaced them with proteins like beans and lentils, tofu, seitan, plant-based meats, nuts, and seeds. You've swapped out cow's milk for nondairy milks like those made from soy, rice, almonds, and coconuts. You've shifted your sweets from the ice cream, cookies, and doughnuts you grew up on to treats sweetened with stevia and agave. Better still, you've taken up eating good old wholesome fruit. And hopefully you've integrated more whole grains into your daily rotation, like brown rice, quinoa, and barley rather than processed white flour and the convenience foods made from it.

On the subject of grains, the Harvard School of Public Health says this when talking about the new U.S. Dietary Guidelines: "Though the new guidelines encourage Americans to cut back on refined grains and replace them with whole grains, they still suggest that it is okay to consume up to half of our grains as refined grains. That's unfortunate, since there's been even more research evidence in the past five years that refined grains, such as white bread, white rice, and white pasta, have adverse metabolic effects and increase the risks of diabetes and heart disease." The Department of Nutrition at Harvard says that refined grains should be used "sparingly, if at all." (Remember, whole grain pastas made from brown rice or quinoa are just fine!)

This is a lot to think about and work out, I know. Everywhere you look, there are advertisements and commercials showing happy people eating fast food, meat, dairy and eggs, and processed junk. I know you join me in looking forward to the day when business establishments and schools provide truly healthy foods, free of all that unneeded fat and sugar that is currently on the menus, and full of all the phytonutrients our bodies crave. They would do well to make that wholesome food available, as the employees and students would surely thrive.

But, alas. You are early on this curve. Give yourself a big pat on the back, and also give yourself some room to figure it all out. We are not quite at that point in history where the demand intersects with supply, so you've got to try a little harder than other people who are not on this path.

Folks doing the Atkins-style diets have no problem finding broiled skinless chicken breasts or pork rinds, for that matter. Animal products are ubiquitous, so these dieters have a much easier go of it than you do. And I would imagine the followers of that kind of eating are grateful to be told (by so-called diet gurus and sponsored research) that they can keep eating what they already have a taste for anyway: "Steaks are good for us? Terrific; this is the diet for me!" But you know the health implications from eating that way (from heart disease to certain types of cancer to type 2 diabetes, and so on), and you have seen the fallout for the creatures who bear the burden of supplying that demand.

Change can be the most natural and easy thing when you feel ready and motivated, while at other times it might feel hard and off-putting, and you find yourself grasping for ways that you can balance everything. Surely, it's never a straight line. Change—especially in an area so elemental as what you eat—comes in fits and starts, going forward and then falling back a bit. But forward you are going! I like what my friend Dr. Dean Ornish says about the process of finding your way: "You have a spectrum of choices; it's not all or nothing. In our research, we learned something very powerful: the more you change, the better you feel and the more you heal. What's sustainable is joy, pleasure, and freedom. If you go *on* a diet, sooner or later you're likely to go *off* a diet—because a diet is what you can't have and what you must do.

"Even more than feeling healthy, most people want to feel free and in control. What matters most is your overall way of living and eating. If you indulge yourself one day, then eat healthier the next, if you forget to exercise or meditate one day, do more the next."

If you are nudging yourself forward, holding to your intention to reshape cravings and habits, you are absolutely moving steadily toward your ideal weight. You might be pleasantly surprised at how swiftly this process carries you.

Eating consciously, moving your body, and doing inner work puts you on track with that evolutionary impulse to transcend who you were before and be your very best. When you focus on living a life that is meaningful and purposeful, everything will fall into that jet stream. You will feel powered up when you think of how much ground you've covered, how much you've grown (and shed!) and overcome.

Take a look around: it seems these days that we are at a critical time in history, where big things can—and need to—really happen. The way we grow and produce food is a tremendous burden on the environment and, as a result of too many people indulging in bad food, an unsustainable burden on the health care system. I want to be part of the change in the way we approach eating. I know you do, too. And as we continue to push ourselves past our less-than-perfect habits and gnawing addictions, we will feel a little stronger each day, a little more empowered knowing that our choices will ripple out and cause a cultural and food revolution. Because really, it's time.

Keep leaning in. Continue to make progress, and don't worry about perfection. Enjoy the ride and keep me posted on your weight loss stories. Your stories make my heart soar, and they change our world, one little bite at a time. Your stories are the revolution.

Here, again, is your list to carry forward:

- ✓ Drink lots of water.
- ✓ Eat a hearty breakfast.
- ✓ Eat an apple.
- ✓ Just for today, say no to your poison.
- ✓ Go a little nuts.
- ✓ Trade up the milk and butter.
- ✓ Put a little flax on it.
- ✓ Do a deep dive for five.
- ✓ Switch up your drinks.
- ✓ Make lunch without animal products.
- ✓ Take your vites.
- ✓ Add in some exercise.
- ✓ Change up your cheese.
- ✓ Eat a superfood.
- ✓ Love yourself a little.
- ✓ Toss up a big bowl of salad.
- ✓ Opt for cashew cream (if it's creaminess you need).
- ✓ Take the animals off the dinner plate.
- ✓ Have a little fun!

✓ Pump it up.
✓ Connect the dots about where food comes from.
✓ Blend up a Power Smoothie.
✓ Back away from sugar.
✓ Visualize your weight loss.
✓ Juice it!
✓ Cut the oil.
✓ Eat lower on the glycemic index.
✓ Do something purposeful.
✓ Schedule your day.
✓ Make progress, and don't worry about perfection.

APPENDIX

What to Eat

THERE IS SO, SO MUCH DELICIOUS FOOD YOU CAN ENJOY WHILE LEANING in. So many scrumptious dishes that just so happen to be healthy, too. In fact, you are likely going to see that your menus will be much more diverse than what you are used to. For instance, you might be used to the same old boring chicken and rice or steak and potatoes, but now you might enjoy the much more tasty black bean cakes with mango salsa or pasta with cashew cream sauce and veggie sausage, all with big colorful salads on the side.

See? Nothing ho-hum for you! And by the way, you can have your chicken and rice, too, if that's what you want, but simply opt for the nonanimal version of chicken and make it brown rice rather than refined white. You'll feel much more satisfied with all that fiber in your system, even while your metabolism is revving up and the pounds are melting off.

I want you to be happy; I want you to feel completely satiated as you explore this wonderful new territory you've leaned into.

I'm going to give you some specific ideas for meals shortly, but in the meantime, I thought this chart from the Physicians Committee for Responsible Medicine (pcrm.org) might help make things clearer for you as you start planning your meals.

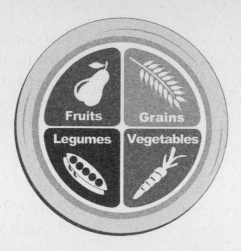

Just think about there being four categories of food: Fruits, Grains (tubers like sweet potatoes and yams are in this category, too, as is whole grain pasta), Legumes (beans, lentils, nuts and seeds, and meat alternatives like veggie burgers are included in this category, too), and Vegetables. As you plan your food for the day, try to hit each food group. Mix it up and try new things, always making sure you are getting your protein (legumes have lots of protein) and veggies, and not just focusing on grains alone.

As the good doctors at PCRM put it, "These four food groups provide the good nutrition you need. There is no need for animal-derived products in the diet, and you're better off without them. Be sure to include a reliable source of vitamin B_{12}, such as any common multiple vitamin or fortified foods."

Fruits

Fruits are rich in fiber, vitamin C, and beta-carotene. Choose a variety of colors, whether fresh or frozen.

Be sure to include at least one serving each day of fruits that are high in vitamin C: citrus fruits, melons, and strawberries are all good choices. (Eat your apple!)

Choose whole fruit over fruit juices, which do not contain very much fiber.

Grains

Grains include bread, rice, pasta, hot or cold cereal, corn, millet, barley, bulgur, buckwheat groats, and tortillas. Build each of your meals around a hearty grain dish—grains are rich in fiber and other complex carbohydrates, as well as protein, B vitamins, and zinc.

Eat more whole grains, such as brown rice, rolled oats, and barley.

Legumes

Legumes—another name for beans, peas, and lentils—are a good source of fiber, protein, iron, calcium, zinc, and B vitamins. This group also includes chickpeas, baked and refried beans, soy milk, tempeh, and tofu. Choose a variety of colors, whether dried, frozen, or canned. (Nuts and nut milks are good, too!)

Vegetables

Vegetables are packed with nutrients. Include generous portions of a variety of vegetables in your diet. Choose a variety of colors, whether fresh, frozen, or canned. They provide vitamin C, beta-carotene, riboflavin, iron, calcium, fiber, and other nutrients.

Dark green leafy vegetables, such as broccoli, collards, kale, mustard and turnip greens, chicory, and bok choy, are especially good sources of these important nutrients.

Dark yellow and orange vegetables, such as carrots, winter squash, sweet potatoes, and pumpkin, provide extra beta-carotene.

And don't forget your superfoods!

Okay, but what does a typical week actually look like, I hear you asking? In my home, it might go something like this . . .

MONDAY

Breakfast: brown rice with chopped walnuts and sliced strawberries and hot nondairy milk on top

Lunch: quinoa with veggies and chickpeas; butternut squash soup

Dinner: stuffed acorn squash with basmati rice, tofu, veggies; big salad (throw everything into salad: chickpeas, nuts, goji berries, raspberries, different lettuces, radishes, tomatoes . . .) with vinaigrette or nondairy creamy dressing

TUESDAY

Breakfast 2: rye toast; peanut or almond butter

Lunch 2: lentil soup; big salad

Dinner 2: tostada with black beans, salsa, sliced avocado; salad

WEDNESDAY

Breakfast 3: steel-cut oatmeal (soaked overnight, heated in the morning), chopped apples, flax, walnuts, hot or cold nondairy milk on top

Lunch 3: seitan Parmesan (slice of nondairy cheese or little bit of Daiya cheese melted on top); tomato sauce; salad

Dinner 3: black bean cakes with mango salsa; basmati rice; green veggies

THURSDAY

Breakfast 4: quinoa (hot or cold); chopped fruit; flax; nondairy milk (cold or steamed)

Lunch 4: whole grain pasta made from brown rice or quinoa; meatless meat crumbles; tomato sauce with veggies mixed in; salad

Dinner 4: Field Roast sausages and sauerkraut; thick vegetable stew

FRIDAY

Breakfast 5: brown rice (it's my favorite!); cinnamon; flax; steamed nondairy milk

Lunch 5: chili with beans and meatless meat crumbles; salad

Dinner 5: portobello mushroom steaks; roasted brussels sprouts; baked sweet potato

SATURDAY

Breakfast 6: scrambled tofu (add turmeric for color); tempeh bacon; rice bread toasted with a touch of Earth Balance nondairy butter on top

Lunch 6: Mediterranean platter of hummus, baba ghanoush, tabbouleh; pita bread; olives

Dinner 6: Italian white beans (a.k.a. cannellini) with rosemary; roasted yams; braised broccolini or greens; salad

SUNDAY

Breakfast 7: manna bread, toasted; peanut or almond butter on top

Lunch 7: veggie burger; nondairy cheese slice; kale salad with walnuts

Dinner 7: Thai curry with tofu and vegetables; salad

It doesn't sound so foreign or difficult when you look at it laid out like that, now does it? You'll hit your stride soon enough when you find a good rotation of favorite meals. Just think of how you used to eat before; you probably had around seven meals that you knew you liked and were easy to prepare. Well, that's what you'll do on the Lean plan, too. You'll try some different foods and experiment with menus, and you'll end up finding the ones that you and your family love, and *voilà*! New habits will be made, just healthier, upgraded ones!

Okay, so now for a few super-simple desserts. Have a dessert one or two nights a week, but not every night (once you get out of the dessert habit, you won't even crave the sweets at all, except for special occasions where tradition calls!). A few ideas that are my faves:

DESSERTS

Baked apple with crumbled nuts on top, a drizzle of agave
    nectar

Bowl of brown rice; half a handful of raisins or currants; steamed Silk Vanilla soy creamer poured over (rice pudding!)

A couple of squares of bittersweet raw chocolate

SNACKS

Some easy, go-to snacks:

Bowl of blueberries with rice or almond milk poured on top

Rice cake with almond butter (spread lightly)

Hummus and carrots, cucumbers

Soy or coconut yogurt with a few seeds and nuts

Handful of goji berries with nuts or seeds

Green juice (kale or collards, celery, cucumber, lemon with rind, ginger, carrots, parsley, mint leaves)

Power Smoothie (recipe on page 164)

Bliss bar (order online)

SunFoods snack bar (order online)

Clif Builders bar (low glycemic index, 20 grams of protein)

PureFit Bar

Vega Bar

Visit the "raw" section of your local health food store and you'll find plenty of yummy treats.

Extra Lean: Eat at home! A *Consumer Reports* survey found that eating at home was one of the most effective habits for losing weight. There are so many hidden calories and fats when you eat out; you'll have better control when you prepare the food yourself. It doesn't have to be fancy, nor does it need to take a long time: a simple bean, veggie, and grain will do. Or a whole grain pasta with veggies and chickpeas with some salad on the side. Even burritos are quick and filling.

If you are like me, you sometimes go out to eat more than you'd like to. Maybe it's a time thing or a business dinner. Whatever the reason, you find yourself in restaurants a lot. Try to avoid this, if at all possible. Cooking at home is the very best way to control what's going into your food, and the time spent at home with your family will be well worth it. Plus, you'll save a ton of money! Start off simply and you'll find it's easier than you think. You can buy canned beans and use frozen cooked brown rice to make quick tacos, or add frozen veggies to that for a hearty bowl of goodies from the power plate.

But in the meantime, here is what you can trend toward when going out:

- Thai, Chinese, or Japanese: edamame, tofu, rice, and all kinds of veggies. If Chinese, steer clear of all those sweet sauces, and keep it simple.
- Mexican: corn fajita (the white flour ones sometimes have lard in them) with black beans, salsa and rice (chips have too much oil).
- Middle Eastern, Greek, or Ethiopian: hummus and baba ghanoush.
- Indian: lentils, chickpeas, and curries (not the ones with cream) with whole grain breads. Ask for dishes made without ghee (clarified butter).
- Pizza places or Italian: pasta (whole grain if they have it) with veggies or spicy tomato sauce; white beans, fava beans, roasted potatoes; salads; pizza with whole grain crust, veggies and onions on top, hold the cheese (sometimes I bring my own nondairy cheese and the pizza maker will use it to make me a super delish vegan cheese pizza).
- Salad bar: lettuces, veggies, chickpeas, olives, mushrooms, tofu, seeds (very light on the vinaigrette!). A side of vegan soup if it's available.

- Burger joints: veggie burgers, without mayo, and with a nice big salad rather than the fries. Baked potato and veggies; salsa or tomato sauce.
- Hotels: ask for oatmeal cooked with water rather than milk; plate of berries; toast and peanut butter (I travel with my own so I know it doesn't have sugar); baked potato, veggies, any kind of beans or legumes they have; minestrone.

If you are on the road, carry some snacks like protein bars or a baggie of nuts and goji berries. You don't want to find yourself starving with nothing to eat and a fast-food joint calling your name!

Okay, so those are the basics. Now for the fun stuff.

Meet Dayna McLeod, a wonderful chef I met a couple of years ago. Dayna wanted to learn how to cook healthy food that both her Australian, meat-loving husband and four-year-old daughter would like, so she attended culinary classes to learn the essentials. And then she took what she learned and started converting her tried-and-true faves from all her travels around the world so that all the dishes were just healthier versions of what she and her family already loved. She turned her favorite recipes into ones without meat, dairy, eggs, or sugar, and I must say, she's done a brilliant job.

Her recipes are simple and practical, and unbelievably delicious, and she's sharing them with you here. Feel free to mix up the main dishes—some you'll want for lunch, others for dinner. There are a few that are one-dish meals, while to others you'll want to add a side dish of a veggie and/or a yam and salad. Dayna will give you some cooking tips along the way, and you'll hear why she loves the dishes she presents here. All that said, feel free to make the dishes your own and experiment until you find what makes your taste buds happiest!

Don't be put off by the long ingredients lists on some of the recipes. These recipes are simple to prepare and simply fantastic.

BREAKFAST

1. BREAKFAST QUINOA

This breakfast quinoa recipe is so delicious it can double as a dessert. Quinoa is naturally loaded with protein and fiber, so it provides long-lasting energy throughout your day. A perfect way to start your morning out right.

Serves 2
Active time: 10 minutes
Start to finish: 25 minutes

Ingredients

½ cup quinoa, rinsed and drained
½ cup unsweetened vanilla almond milk
½ cup water
Pinch salt
1 teaspoon Earth Balance spread
1 medium apple, diced, with peel
1 teaspoon ground cinnamon
¼ cup chopped toasted walnuts
1 tablespoon agave nectar

1. In a small saucepan, bring the quinoa, milk, water, and salt to a boil for 2 minutes.
2. Reduce, heat to low and cover for 15 minutes or until all the water is absorbed. Remove from the heat and let sit, covered, for 5 minutes.
3. Meanwhile, in a small skillet over medium heat, melt the Earth Balance spread. Add the apple, stir together until evenly coated, and sauté for 1 minute. Cover and cook for 3 minutes, or until soft
4. Add the cinnamon and walnuts and cook for 1 additional minute.
5. Stir in the apple mixture with the quinoa, and divide between two bowls.
6. Drizzle the agave nectar on top and enjoy!

****Helpful Hint**** Quinoa is a South American grain that needs to be rinsed well before cooking. Quinoa has a natural coating that can make the cooked grains bitter and mushy if they are not washed first.

****Variations**** For a simple change, cook the quinoa as directed above, but omit the apple and Earth Balance spread. Gently fold blackberries and cinnamon into the quinoa, and top with walnuts, agave nectar, and shredded coconut.

2. PUMPKIN FLAPJACKS

Pumpkin gives a traditional pancake a sweet, surprising twist. Adding ginger and cinnamon completes the transformation from ordinary to extraordinary!

Serves 4
Active time: 10 minutes
Start to finish: 20 minutes

Ingredients

- 1 cup gluten-free flour (I like Bob's Red Mill brand)
- ½ teaspoon salt
- 2 teaspoons baking powder
- ¼ teaspoon allspice
- ⅛ teaspoon ground cloves
- 1 teaspoon ground ginger
- 1 teaspoon ground cinnamon
- ¼ teaspoon ground nutmeg
- 1 cup pumpkin, canned or pureed fresh
- 1 cup almond milk
- ½ cup water
- 2 tablespoons vegetable oil
- 2 tablespoons agave nectar
- 2 teaspoons apple cider vinegar
- 1 teaspoon vanilla extract

Cooking spray
Toasted pecans for garnish

1. Sift the flour, salt and baking powder together in a large bowl. Add the spices and mix well.
2. In a separate bowl, whisk together the pumpkin, milk, water, oil, agave nectar, vinegar, and vanilla.
3. Fold the pumpkin mixture into the dry ingredients.
4. Preheat a large, seasoned cast-iron skillet over medium heat for 5 minutes.
5. Spray the pan with a small amount of cooking spray.
6. Pour ¼ cup of batter for each pancake.
7. Cook the pancakes about 3 minutes per side, or until golden brown.
8. Garnish with pecans and serve immediately.

****For Your Information****The pumpkin does make the pancakes a bit dense. They will taste and feel heavier than a plain pancake. Don't be alarmed! More importantly, don't be deterred from making these delicious flapjacks!
****Buy and Try**** Look for Bob's Red Mill brand products the next time you are at the store. They have some fantastic, healthy baking ingredients that I just love to use while cooking. You can also order their products through Amazon.com.

DRESSINGS, SPREADS, AND DIPS

1. CLASSIC HUMMUS

Hummus is a nutritional treasure. It's not only delicious to eat, it is packed with protein and contains lots of vitamins, minerals, omega-3s, and amino acids. This amazing authentic Mediterranean recipe was given to me from my friends at Baba Foods SLO.

Serves 4
Active time: 5 minutes
Start to finish: 10 minutes

Ingredients

> 3 tablespoons tahini
> 3 tablespoons lemon juice
> 2 (15 oz.) cans garbanzo beans, rinsed and drained
> 1 clove garlic, chopped
> 1 tablespoon water
> 1 tablespoon olive oil
> Dash salt
> Dash pepper
> Pinch cumin powder or ground cumin

1. In a small bowl, mix the tahini and lemon juice.
2. In a food processor, combine the garbanzos, garlic, and water, and blend until smooth.
3. Slowly add in the tahini and lemon juice mixture while continuing to blend.
4. Then slowly add in the olive oil, salt, pepper, and cumin.
5. Continue blending until the mixture is extremely smooth.
6. Taste and add seasoning if needed.

****Variation**** This Mediterranean dip lends itself to several variations. Here are just a few flavors you can make: sun-dried tomato, spicy black bean, basil pesto, roasted red pepper, dill and mint, cilantro and avocado, jalapeño, Kalamata olive, artichoke, and roasted garlic . . . and the list goes on and on.
****Serving Ideas**** Serve with flatbread, use as a dip for a vegetable crudité, use it in a wrap, serve it with warm pita triangles, or even on top of a salad to add some protein.

2. GUACAMOLE

This recipe is just a base for your guacamole creation; feel free to improvise. Any way you mash it, it is an easy way to dress up a dish. Fun to bring to a party!

Serves 4
Active time: 10 minutes
Start to finish: 10 minutes

Ingredients

    2 large ripe avocados, peeled and pitted
    1 medium Roma tomato, seeded and diced
    3 green onions, chopped
    1 teaspoon minced fresh red jalapeño pepper
    ¼ teaspoon cumin powder
    ⅓ cup fresh roughly chopped cilantro
    2 tablespoons fresh lime juice
    Salt and pepper to taste

1. Scoop out the avocado flesh and place in a medium bowl. Mash with a fork, being careful not to overdo it, to preserve some small chunks.
2. Add the tomato, onions, jalapeño, cumin, and cilantro, and combine.
3. Squeeze in the lime juice, and season with salt and pepper.

****Helpful Hint**** While storing in the refrigerator, keep your guacamole from turning brown by placing a layer of plastic kitchen wrap directly on the guacamole surface and squeeze out the air.
****Chef's Secret**** For extra spicy guacamole, leave the jalapeño seeds in your mix!
****Serving Suggestions**** Serve this with your terrific tacos, or serve as a dip with some healthy corn chips.

3. PRESTO PESTO

I call this recipe Presto Pesto because it is so simple you can make it in a matter of minutes. This recipe uses just seven ingredients and makes a sauce packed full of flavor!

Serves 10
Active time: 10 minutes
Start to finish: 10 minutes

Ingredients

1¼ cups toasted pine nuts
2 bunches fresh basil leaves
1 cup olive oil
2 cloves garlic, chopped
¼ teaspoon freshly ground black pepper
¼ teaspoon salt
1 teaspoon lemon juice

1. To toast the pine nuts, preheat your toaster oven to 350°F. Spread the nuts on the toasting pan and bake until lightly brown, about 4 minutes. Shake the pan once or twice midway through cooking for even toasting.
2. Prepare a bowl of ice water. Bring a large pot of water to a boil.
3. Gather all the basil leaves, making sure to discard the stalks.
4. Plunge the basil into the boiling water for 10 seconds, making sure all the leaves are pushed under the water. Drain the pot and plunge the basil into the ice water to stop the cooking. Squeeze the basil of all excess water and lay the basil on a paper towel.
5. In a food processor, pulse all the ingredients together (including the toasted nuts).
6. Season to taste.

****Variation**** This recipe calls for pine nuts. You could certainly substitute cashews if you'd prefer. They are definitely the less expensive option of the two.
****Serving Ideas**** Pesto is so versatile; you'll never run out of ways to enjoy it. You can toss it with pasta, use it as a sandwich

spread, make pizza sauce, even just serve it with crackers for an appetizer.

*****Time-saving Tip****Make a double batch of this recipe and store it in a sealed jar for up to 2 weeks. You can even freeze it in ice cube trays and use it next month.

4. RANCH DRESSING

When I was considering cutting out dairy, one of my first thoughts was, how would I live without ranch dressing? Ranch dressing is about as American as apple pie. Needless to say, this was the first recipe I decided to perfect, and it doesn't disappoint.

Serves 8
Active time: 10 minutes
Start to finish: 2 hours, 10 minutes

Ingredients

> 5 ounces firm silken-style tofu, drained (I like Mori-Nu brand)
> ½ cup light vegan mayonnaise (I like Reduced Fat Vegenaise brand)
> 2 tablespoons freshly squeezed lemon juice
> ⅓ cup unsweetened soy milk
> 1 teaspoon minced or pressed garlic
> 1 teaspoon minced shallot
> 3 green onions, sliced
> 1 tablespoon roughly chopped fresh dill
> 1 teaspoon vegan Worcestershire sauce
> 2 teaspoons Dijon-style mustard
> 1 teaspoon onion powder
> ½ teaspoon celery seed powder
> ¼ teaspoon salt
> ¼ teaspoon freshly ground black pepper
> 2 tablespoons roughly chopped fresh chives

1. In a blender or food processor, combine all the ingredients except the chives.
2. Mix until you have a smooth and creamy sauce.
3. Add the fresh chives to the mix, and pulse one time, keeping the chives in larger pieces.
4. This dressing should be chilled for 2 hours before serving.

****Helpful Hint**** Refrigerate overnight in a sealed jar to enjoy a more robust flavor.

****Serving Ideas**** Ranch is not just for salad anymore! You can use this creamy delight on just about anything. Pour it over a baked potato, use it as a yummy sandwich spread, or use it as a dip for anything your imagination can think of.

5. CREAMY AVOCADO DRESSING

A great salad deserves a great dressing. With ingredients so fresh, this one blends beautifully with any salad you choose. Did you know avocados are high in fiber? So not only do they taste unbelievable, but they help fill you up.

Serves 4
Active time: 10 minutes
Start to finish: 10 minutes

Ingredients

> 2 cloves garlic, minced or pressed
> 1 ripe avocado, pitted and peeled
> ¼ cup minced fresh cilantro
> 1½ tablespoons fresh lime juice
> 1 teaspoon agave nectar
> 1 teaspoon rice vinegar
> 2 tablespoons water
> ½ teaspoon salt

⅛ teaspoon ground cayenne pepper
¼ cup olive oil

1. Combine the garlic, avocado, cilantro, lime juice, agave, vinegar, water, salt, and cayenne, and blend well in a food processor.
2. Continue to blend as you slowly pour a thin stream of olive oil through the opening in the top of the food processor. Blend until smooth and creamy.

****For Your Information**** This salad dressing should be made and used the same day.

MAIN COURSES

1. BLACK BEAN SALSA SALAD

Warning! This dish is highly addictive. This recipe dates back to the 1950s and was created by a famous chef at Neiman Marcus. Sixty-one years later I have adapted this mouthwatering dish into a healthier version. Make copies of this recipe because people always ask for it.

Serves 6
Active time: 10 minutes
Start to finish: 1 hour, 10 minutes

Ingredients

2 (16 oz.) cans black beans, drained but not rinsed
1 (14 oz.) can fire-roasted diced tomatoes with green chiles (or similar), drained but not rinsed
1 (8 oz.) can small white shoepeg corn
½ cup broccoli florets, chopped into small florets
½ bunch green onions, diced small
½ English cucumber, seeded and diced

2 stalks celery, chopped into ¼-inch dice
1 red bell pepper, diced small
1 yellow bell pepper, diced small
1 green pepper, diced small
1 bunch fresh cilantro leaves, chopped
1 tablespoon olive oil
1 lime, squeezed
¼ cup wine vinegar
1 clove garlic, minced or pressed
1 teaspoon cumin powder
Salt and pepper to taste
1 avocado, diced small
Salad greens

1. Combine the beans, vegetables, and cilantro in a large bowl.
2. In a separate small bowl, whisk together the oil, lime juice, vinegar, garlic, cumin, and salt and pepper.
3. Pour the dressing on top of the bean mixture and toss to coat.
4. Cover and chill for an hour or overnight to allow the flavors to develop.
5. Dice the avocado and combine immediately before serving. Plate on top of salad greens.

****Helpful Hint**** This is a perfect dish to bring to a party. To serve it as a dip, omit the broccoli, celery, cucumbers, and avocado. Serve dip with blue corn chips and you will have a real crowd-pleaser. Every party has some sort of salad. Grab some greens from the salad and pour this mixture on top. *Voilà* . . . you now have your main course.

2. BEST BEEFLESS BURGER IN TOWN

Mmmm . . . burgers. They're not just for meat lovers anymore! So fire up your grill, and get ready for one of these thick, juicy homemade burgers. They are sure to be a hit at your next cookout!

Serves 2
Active time: 10 minutes
Start to finish: 20 minutes

Ingredients

⅓ cup tamari soy sauce

2 tablespoons olive oil

2 Gardein Beefless Burgers, frozen

2 tablespoons light vegan mayonnaise (I like
   Vegenaise)

1 tablespoon ketchup

1 tablespoon sweet relish

Garlic powder to taste

2 slices vegan Cheddar cheese, sliced

2 multigrain sandwich thins, toasted

4 lettuce leaves

1 tomato, sliced

½ small red onion, slices

½ small avocado, slices

1. Combine the soy sauce and olive oil and marinate the patties in a small ziplock bag for 5 minutes in the refrigerator.
2. In the meantime, make the dressing. Combine the Vegenaise, ketchup, and relish in a small bowl and mix well.
3. Sprinkle each frozen patty with a light, even coat of garlic powder.
4. Preheat the grill to medium heat.
5. Grill the burgers for 4 minutes per side, or until each patty is nice and brown.
6. Top with a slice of Cheddar cheese in the last minute of cooking, and cover to melt.
7. Toast the sandwich thins for 1–2 minutes on the grill.

8. Remove from the heat and spread the dressing on the insides of the sandwich thins.
9. Place a cheeseburger on each thin, and stack your toppings and enjoy!

****Healthy Tip**** Trying to reduce your carb intake? Skip the sandwich thin and wrap cold crisp lettuce around your burger. Romaine and iceberg lettuce seem to work best.

****Variation**** The sky is the limit for toppings on your burger. Whether it's grilled wild mushrooms, tempeh bacon, soy blue cheese crumbles, grilled pineapple, roasted balsamic onions, jerk seasoning, red beetroot, pickles, salsa, horseradish, roasted red peppers, sun-dried tomatoes . . . the list goes on and on!

3. COCONUT GARBANZO BEAN CURRY

This savory garbanzo bean curry is delicious served over couscous. If there is any left over, pack it in a thermos and take it to work for lunch the next day. This dish travels well, and the flavor actually intensifies overnight!

Serves 4
Active time: 35 minutes
Start to finish: 45 minutes

Ingredients

1 cup butternut squash, peeled and cut into ½-inch cubes
1 cup sweet potato, peeled and cut into ½-inch cubes
2 tablespoons olive oil
1 medium yellow onion, chopped
1 medium red bell pepper, cut in ¼-inch dice
1 tablespoon African curry powder (or other favorite curry powder)
3 cloves garlic, minced or pressed

2 tablespoons creamy peanut butter

1 can lite unsweetened coconut milk

1 (14 oz.) can diced tomatoes, drained

2 (15 oz.) cans garbanzo beans, drained and rinsed

¼ teaspoon freshly ground black pepper

¼ teaspoon salt

4 cups fresh spinach

2 tablespoons roughly chopped fresh cilantro

¼ cup chopped unsalted roasted peanuts

1. Preheat oven to 425°F.
2. Toss the squash and sweet potato cubes in a medium bowl with 1 tablespoon of olive oil until the cubes are evenly coated. Place the squash and potatoes in a single layer on a roasting pan or baking sheet. Roast for 20–30 minutes, or until soft in the middle.
3. In the meantime, heat 1 tablespoon of olive oil in a large saucepan over medium heat. Add the onion and bell pepper and sauté until soft, 5–8 minutes.
4. Add the curry powder and garlic, and stir constantly for 30 seconds.
5. Stir in the peanut butter and slowly add the coconut milk until a very smooth sauce is formed.
6. Add in the tomatoes, garbanzo beans, sweet potatoes, and squash, and mix until combined.
7. Season with the pepper and salt and bring the mixture up to a simmer. Stir in the spinach until wilted, about 5 minutes.
8. Stir in the cilantro and remove from the heat. Top with the peanuts before serving.

****Did You Know**** Some studies have shown that ingredients in curry may help to prevent certain diseases, including colon cancer and Alzheimer's disease. Curry powders are extremely diverse: some red, some yellow, some brown, some with five spices and some with as many as 20 or more. While curry powder can be bought at

any grocery store, you may want to broaden your palate by finding
more at a specialty store. I bought this particular African curry powder at Williams-Sonoma. World Market and other online shops are
of course great alternatives.

4. COLD SOBA NOODLE SALAD
WITH PEANUT DRESSING

This fantastic salad is filled with fiber and protein, and is bursting
with flavor! Soba is chock-full of a potent antioxidant called rutin.
It has been shown to improve circulation and prevent LDL cholesterol from clogging blood vessels.

Serves 4
Active time: 30 minutes
Start to finish: 45 minutes

Ingredients

   14 ounces extra-firm tofu, pressed and drained
   2 tablespoons low-sodium tamari soy sauce
   2 teaspoons toasted sesame oil
   ⅓ cup brown rice vinegar
   ⅔ cup creamy peanut butter
   ¼ cup agave nectar
   ¼ cup orange juice
   2 cloves garlic
   1 tablespoon peeled and minced fresh gingerroot
   ¼ cup water
   ⅛ teaspoon crushed red pepper flakes
   1 cup fresh cilantro leaves
   1 bag soba noodles
   1 tablespoon toasted sesame oil
   ½ cucumber, diced
   2 carrots, julienned

3 green onions, sliced
1 red bell pepper, thinly sliced
¼ cup shredded red cabbage
⅓ cup frozen edamame, defrosted and shelled
⅓ cup bean sprouts
½ can water chestnuts, sliced
1 head lettuce leaves
Toasted slivered almonds

1. Cut the pressed tofu into ½-inch cubes. A simple technique to do this is to cut the tofu block in half. Now cut those 2 halves into halves. Rotate the block 90 degrees and repeat.
2. Combine the tamari, sesame oil, vinegar, peanut butter, agave nectar, orange juice, garlic, ginger, water, and red pepper flakes in a blender or food processor until creamy.
3. Add the cilantro and pulse, being careful not to overblend. The cilantro should look chopped.
4. Using a small amount of the dressing as a marinade, cover the tofu in a shallow container. Chill and marinate the tofu for at least 20 minutes. At this time, you can also chill the remainder of the dressing for your salad.
5. In a large pot of boiling water, cook soba noodles for 5 minutes, or until al dente. You may need to turn down the heat to bring the water to a slow boil. Soba makes froth on top of the water and may quickly overflow your pot.
6. Drain and rinse the noodles well in cold water. Put the noodles in a container with a top, and toss the noodles with 1 tablespoon of toasted sesame oil. This helps prevent the noodles from sticking. Chill the noodles for at least 15 minutes.
7. Meanwhile, combine all the vegetables in a very large bowl.
8. Transfer the cold noodles and dressing into the same bowl, and toss well to coat.
9. Place a few lettuce leaves on each plate. Using tongs, divide the noodle mixture among the four plates on top of the greens.

10. Arrange the tofu pieces around the noodles.
11. Garnish with toasted slivered almonds.

****Chef's Secret**** Many vegan recipes call for pressed tofu. This simple process removes excess moisture, allowing more flavor to be absorbed while cooking. The easiest way I have found to do it is as follows:

1. Remove the tofu from the container and drain the water in a colander over the sink.
2. Layer 2 clean kitchen towels on top of a cutting board.
3. Lay the tofu block on the towels, and lay three more clean towels on top of the tofu.
4. Carefully lay another cutting board on top of the towels.
5. Place 2 heavy books or soup cans on top of the cutting board.
6. Let sit for at least 20 minutes.

****Variation**** Use whatever vegetables you have in the refrigerator for this salad. The great thing about cooking is you can tailor each recipe to fit your needs!

5. GREEK SALAD

A traditional Greek salad features tomatoes, cucumbers, and olives, but this mouthwatering recipe takes the concept to a whole different level. You and your taste buds will be thanking the Greek gods after just one bite.

Serves 2
Active time: 15 minutes
Start to finish: 15 minutes

Ingredients

2 cups chopped romaine lettuce
1 small English cucumber, seeded and diced

6 whole sun-dried tomatoes, drained and diced

¼ small red onion, diced

10 whole Kalamata olives, pitted and drained

4 whole canned artichoke hearts in water, drained and
    halved

½ cup crumbled vegan soy feta

½ cup olive oil

¼ cup lemon juice

2 cloves garlic, minced or pressed

2 teaspoons dried oregano

1 teaspoon dried basil

1 tablespoon finely chopped fresh dill

2 tablespoons red wine vinegar

1 tablespoon agave nectar

2 tablespoons water

½ teaspoon salt

¼ teaspoon freshly ground black pepper

2 whole peperoncini peppers, drained

1. In a large bowl, mix all the vegetables and the feta together. Set aside while you make the vinaigrette.
2. In a small bowl, whisk together the oil, lemon juice, garlic, oregano, basil, dill, vinegar, agave, water, and salt and pepper.
3. Pour over the salad and toss to combine the herb vinaigrette with the vegetables.
4. Garnish with a peperoncini on top. Serve immediately.

****Chef's Secret**** The secret to this scrumptious salad is to dice the vegetables to the same size so that the flavors can blend into one bite.

****Variations**** For some added protein, you can add in some tofu or quinoa. For some extra nutritional value, cooked barley will do the trick.

****Buy and Try**** Sunergia Soy Foods Soy Feta and Soy Bleu "cheese." If you don't have a large selection of vegan products at your local store, there are great shopping resources online. Even Amazon carries some great products now.

6. HEARTY LENTIL SOUP

This yummy lentil soup recipe is bursting with nourishment from the lentils and an assortment of veggies. This soup is packed with protein and will keep you satisfied all day long. It freezes well and seems to improve with each leftover serving.

Serves 6
Active time: 20 minutes
Start to finish: 1 hour, 20 minutes

Ingredients

> 1 tablespoon olive oil
> 1 medium yellow onion, cut into ¼-inch cubes
> 2 cups Yukon Gold potatoes, cut into ½-inch cubes
> 4 stalks celery, chopped
> 4 carrots, chopped
> 2 leeks, white and light green only, thinly sliced
> 3 cloves garlic, minced or pressed
> 8 cups vegetable stock
> 2 cups brown and/or green lentils, thoroughly rinsed and
>   picked over
> 2 bay leaves
> 2 tablespoons dried parsley
> 1 tablespoon dried basil
> 1 tablespoon dried oregano
> Salt and pepper to taste

1. In a large soup pot, heat the oil over medium heat. Sauté the onion, potatoes, celery, carrots, leeks, and garlic until golden, about 5 minutes.

2. Next pour the vegetable stock into the pot, and add the rinsed lentils, herbs, and salt and pepper to taste.
3. Increase the heat to high and bring the soup to a boil.
4. Cover, reduce the heat to a simmer, and cook for 1 hour.
5. Make sure the level of the stock isn't too low, adding more stock as necessary.
6. Taste and add more salt and pepper if necessary.
7. The soup should be thick and creamy, and the lentils nice and soft.

****Helpful Hint**** Be sure to pick through your lentils carefully. It is easy to find tiny pebbles and grit.
****Buy and Try**** If you are using a store-bought stock, try a brand called Better Than Bouillon. The No Chicken Base is my favorite.

7. MOROCCAN PASTA WITH GARBANZO BEANS

This pasta is a personal favorite of mine. It takes only 30 minutes to make, so it's a great option after a long day at work. This dish is served best cold. Make this recipe ahead of time for a dinner after a long day.

Serves 4
Active time: 15 minutes
Start to finish: 30 minutes

Ingredients

2 tablespoons olive oil
1 medium yellow onion, cut into ¼-inch dice
½ (8 oz.) package rice pasta elbows or spirals (I like
     Tinkyada brand)
3 cloves garlic, minced or pressed
1 teaspoon ground coriander
1 teaspoon cumin powder

1 teaspoon harissa

½ teaspoon ground allspice

1 teaspoon finely ground sea salt

¼ teaspoon coarsely ground black pepper

1 (15 oz.) can garbanzo beans, rinsed and drained

1 (28 oz.) can crushed Italian tomatoes

¼ cup chopped fresh Italian parsley, loosely packed

1. Heat the oil in a 3-quart sauté pan over medium-high heat.
2. Add the onion and sauté for 2 minutes, stirring constantly.
3. Reduce the heat to low and cover the pan for 15 minutes, until the onion is translucent.
4. While the onion is cooking, bring a large pot of water to a rapid boil and cook the pasta as directed on the package.
5. When the onion is cooked, add in the garlic, coriander, cumin, harissa, allspice, salt, and pepper, and cook for 1 minute, stirring constantly.
6. Stir in the garbanzo beans and tomatoes and bring to a boil over high heat. Once it has reached a boil, stir, reduce the heat to a simmer, and cover.
7. Drain the pasta and mix in with the tomato sauce, continuing over low heat for 3 minutes. Do not overstir! Too much stirring will cause the pasta to break apart and turn mushy.
8. Sprinkle with the parsley just before serving.

****Helpful Hint**** Cook all rice pasta 3–4 minutes less than directed on package. This will help with the nice al dente effect, and your pasta won't break apart and turn to mush!

****For Your Information**** Harissa is a Tunisian hot chile spice. It is available in most supermarkets in the spice aisle. Harissa can come in a paste form or in dry flakes. Specialty stores will also carry harissa. I know for sure Whole Foods and Williams-Sonoma keep it as a staple item and it's available online and in spice shops.

If you can't find it, substitute ¼ teaspoon crushed red pepper flakes.

8. PHILLY NO STEAK SANDWICH

Being a nonmeat eater is no reason to miss out on the warm goodness of a Philly cheesesteak! This recipe replaces beef with seitan, a protein-filled meat substitute made from wheat gluten.

Serves 2
Active time: 15 minutes
Start to finish: 25 minutes

Ingredients

> 2 tablespoons olive oil
> 1 small onion, cut in half vertically and thinly sliced
> 1 green pepper, sliced
> 1 red pepper, sliced
> 2 cloves garlic, minced or pressed
> 1 (12 oz.) package seitan, finely chopped
> 1 teaspoon vegan Worcestershire sauce
> 1 teaspoon garlic powder
> ⅛ teaspoon freshly ground pepper
> 4 slices vegan provolone cheese (if not available, use
>   vegan mozzarella), torn into strips
> 2 whole wheat sandwich thins
> 1 cup vegan marinara sauce (optional)

1. Heat 1 tablespoon olive oil in a large skillet over medium heat.
2. Sauté the onion and peppers for 3 minutes, stirring occasionally. Cover and reduce the heat to low for 5 minutes, or until the onion becomes soft and translucent.

3. Uncover and increase to medium-high heat. Add the remaining tablespoon of oil, the garlic cloves, and chopped seitan. Make sure all the water is pressed out of the seitan before cooking to keep oil from splattering.
4. Pour the Worcestershire sauce, garlic powder, and pepper over the meat while constantly stirring the meat.
5. Cook for approximately 4 minutes or until the seitan starts to turn golden.
6. Lay the cheese on top of the meat mixture and reduce the heat to low. When the cheese is melted, pile onto the sandwich thins and top with warm marinara sauce if desired.

****Buy and Try**** You can now purchase whole wheat sandwich thins at almost any supermarket. Only 100 calories for the entire bun! You can also substitute Food for Life Ezekiel 4:9 bread, which is always a healthy option.

****Variation**** Replace the seitan with Gardein beefless tips. They are found in your grocer's freezer section.

9. SPAGHETTI BOLOGNESE

Mamma mia! Who doesn't love spaghetti bolognese? Everyone has their own version of this Italian classic, and I have my own, too. I gave this sauce a vegan makeover, and the results are phenomenal! This is comfort food at its best!

Serves 8
Active time: 20 minutes
Start to finish: 45 minutes

Ingredients

2 tablespoons olive oil
1 medium yellow onion, chopped

1 cup sliced mushrooms

3 cloves garlic, minced or pressed

1 package soy crumbles (I like Smart Ground from Lightlife)

1 jar vegan marinara sauce

10 fresh basil leaves, cut into chiffonade

1 package rice pasta, spaghetti noodles

1 red bell pepper, diced

1 green bell pepper, diced

½ cup diced zucchini

½ cup broccoli florets

½ cup cauliflower florets

Salt and pepper to taste

Fresh parsley sprigs for garnish

1. Place a large soup pot over medium heat. Add 1 tablespoon of the oil and heat for 30 seconds.
2. Add the onion and mushrooms and sauté until soft, about 5 minutes. Add the garlic and sauté for 1 minute longer.
3. Add the soy crumbles and stir to combine.
4. Pour the marinara sauce into the pot and stir in the fresh basil.
5. Cover, reduce the heat to low, and simmer for at least 20 minutes, stirring occasionally.
6. Bring a large pot of water to a boil and cook the noodles as directed on the package.
7. Meanwhile, in a large skillet or wok, heat the remaining oil over medium heat.
8. Stir in all the vegetables and sauté, being careful not to overcook. The vegetables should still be a bit crunchy when finished.
9. Transfer the vegetables into the pot with the marinara sauce and stir to combine.
10. Season the sauce with salt and pepper to taste.
11. Drain the noodles and toss together with the sauce. Garnish with the fresh parsley sprigs and serve immediately.

****Helpful Hint**** Chiffonade is a simple technique for cutting basil or mint. Stack several (about 6) basil leaves. Roll the pile of leaves lengthwise into a tight cigar shape. Using a very sharp knife, cut the bundled leaves into thin slices. Fluff the chiffonade with your fingers. You can sprinkle on soups, stir into a dish, or just use it as a garnish to decorate a plate. It's an easy way to impress your guests! ****Chef's Secret**** Substituting the meat with soy crumbles and adding heaps of yummy veggies is a meal in itself. You probably noticed this recipe makes a huge amount of food, and I did that on purpose. This meal freezes great, and may just taste even better the second time around. Some days you just don't have time to cook. By having premade meals readily available, you don't have to reach for junk food anymore.

10. SUNNY CITRUS QUINOA SALAD

This delicious salad is packed with protein and whole grain fiber. Salads are something people either love or hate, and I try to get people to love them by exposing them to salads like this. All salads are not created equal!

Serves 2
Active time: 20 minutes
Start to finish: 40 minutes

Ingredients

> 1 cup quinoa, rinsed and drained
> 2 cups water
> ½ cup orange juice, preferably fresh
> 1 tablespoon minced shallot
> 2 tablespoons chopped fresh cilantro, loosely packed
> 2 tablespoons chopped fresh mint, loosely packed
> 2 tablespoons chopped fresh parsley, loosely packed

1 tablespoon chopped chives
1 teaspoon freshly grated orange zest
1 teaspoon ground coriander
1 teaspoon ground cumin
½ teaspoon salt
¼ teaspoon freshly ground pepper
2 tablespoons olive oil
¼ cup toasted slivered almonds
¼ cup raisins
¼ cup golden raisins
⅓ cup chopped dried apricots
1 head butter lettuce, leaves separated
1 large navel orange, peeled and sectioned

1. Make the quinoa: Rinse well in a fine-mesh strainer until the water is clear. Place the quinoa and 2 cups of water in a small saucepan over high heat. Bring to a boil for 2 minutes. Cover and turn off the heat. Leave covered for 20 minutes, or until all water is absorbed.
2. In the meantime, combine the orange juice, shallot, cilantro, mint, parsley, and chives in a medium bowl.
3. Add the zest, coriander, cumin, salt, and pepper to the orange juice mix. Whisk the olive oil into mixture.
4. Toast the almonds, if desired, in a toaster oven until light brown.
5. Fluff the quinoa with a fork and transfer to a large bowl. Toss in the raisins, apricots, and dressing.
6. Place the lettuce and orange sections onto a plate, and top with the quinoa salad.
7. Sprinkle the toasted almonds on top for garnish.

**** A Helpful Tip**** Did you know quinoa is a great staple that can be used for breakfast, lunch, or dinner? I like to make 2 cups of quinoa at the start of each week. I put it in the refrigerator so I always have protein at my fingertips. This is a great time-saver tip!

11. ULTIMATE BLT SANDWICH

What takes this sandwich from unflavored to ultimate is the addition of the nutrient-dense avocado. This heavenly fruit has 20 essential nutrients and is a rich source of fiber. Not only does it taste wonderful, you'll be satisfied for hours.

Serves 2
Active time: 10 minutes
Start to finish: 20 minutes

Ingredients

>   1 tablespoon olive oil
>   6 pieces tempeh bacon
>   4 slices sprouted-grain bread, toasted lightly
>   4 romaine lettuce leaves
>   4 slices tomatoes
>   6 slices ripe avocado
>   Salt and pepper to taste
>   2 tablespoons light vegan mayonnaise (such as
>   Vegenaise)

1. In a medium sauté pan, heat the oil and cook the bacon according to the package directions. Be sure to watch the bacon closely, as it can burn quickly. Place the cooked strips onto a paper towel–lined plate. Set aside to cool.
2. Lightly toast the bread and spread 2 slices with the Vegenaise.
3. Assemble as you would a BLT, adding avocado on top.
4. Sprinkle salt and pepper to taste.

****Variation**** I like to omit the vegan mayonnaise and instead spread yummy hummus on my bread.

****Buy and Try**** Ezekiel 4:9 Sprouted Grain Bread, Lightlife Fakin Bacon, or Lightlife Smart Bacon

****Helpful Hint**** Packing a vegan BLT sandwich for lunches is easy. Just wrap the sandwich in plastic wrap and put in a cooler. This sandwich travels well and makes for a great office lunch.

12. CHINESE STIR-FRY

Hungry for Chinese food? This budget-friendly recipe is quick and easy, and it tastes delicious over a bed of brown rice. Stir-fries are a simple way to get dinner on the table fast, and you get to show off your chopstick skills.

Serves 2
Active time: 25 minutes
Start to finish: 30 minutes

Ingredients

8 ounces firm or extra-firm tofu, pressed and drained
4 tablespoons mirin
2 tablespoons cornstarch
2 tablespoons low-sodium tamari soy sauce
¼ teaspoon crushed red pepper flakes
1 teaspoon agave
1 teaspoon toasted sesame oil
½ cup orange juice
1 tablespoon canola oil
1 tablespoon fresh gingerroot, peeled and very finely minced
3 cloves garlic, minced or pressed
1 bag frozen stir-fry vegetables

1. Cut the pressed tofu into cubes.
2. In a shallow covered container, whisk together the mirin and cornstarch. Add the tofu cubes, cover, and shake the container to evenly coat the tofu. Marinate for at least 20 minutes.

3. In a small bowl, mix together the tamari, red pepper flakes, agave, sesame oil, and orange juice.
4. Heat the canola oil in a wok over medium-high heat. Add in the ginger and garlic and sauté for 1 minute.
5. Using a slotted spoon, remove the tofu from the marinade and sauté the tofu in the wok. Turn the tofu with tongs or a spatula often. All sides of the tofu should be golden brown.
6. Now toss in the frozen vegetables and the tamari mixture. Cook for about 3–5 minutes, or until your vegetables are done. Remember to stir frequently to prevent burning your food. The wok is extremely hot!

****Helpful Hint**** If you are using fresh vegetables, the cooking of this stir-fry moves quickly, so make sure all your ingredients are chopped and ready to go before you begin.

****Variations**** Use any colorful combination of vegetables you please for this dish. A stir-fry is a great way to incorporate more vegetables into your family's diet.

13. CREAMY PUMPKIN PASTA

Halloween is by far my favorite holiday of the year. One thing I've learned, pumpkins aren't just for decorating anymore. Pumpkin is packed with nutrition, and is an excellent source for vitamin A and fiber. Just one more reason to love Halloween!

Serves 4
Active time: 10 minutes
Start to finish: 25 minutes

Ingredients

> 1 pound rice pasta (I like Tinkyada Spirals), cooked al dente
> 1 tablespoon olive oil

2 links vegan sausage, cut on the bias

1 medium onion, finely chopped

4 cloves garlic, minced or pressed

6 fresh sage leaves, cut into chiffonade

1 bay leaf

½ cup dry white wine

1 cup canned pumpkin

1 cup vegan chicken stock (I like Better than Bouillon
     No Chicken Base)

½ cup cashew cream (see page 120)

⅛ teaspoon ground cinnamon

½ teaspoon ground nutmeg

⅛ teaspoon allspice

Salt and pepper to taste

1. In a large pot over medium-high heat, bring water to a boil for pasta. Cook your pasta according to the package directions.
2. Meanwhile, place a large nonstick skillet over medium-high heat, add the oil to the pan, and brown the sausage (about 3 minutes on each side). Transfer the sausages to a paper towel–lined tray.
3. In a large deep sauté pan, add the remaining tablespoon of oil and bring the heat to medium-high. Sauté the onion for 5 minutes, until translucent and tender. Add the garlic to the onion for an additional minute, continuously stirring to prevent the garlic from burning.
4. Add the sage, bay leaf, and wine to your pan, and reduce by half. This should take only a minute or so. Add the pumpkin and stock, stirring continuously to combine. Increase the heat to high and bring to a boil. Stir in the cashew cream, return your sausage to the pan, and reduce the heat to low. Add the spices to the sauce and simmer for 5–10 minutes, or until the sauce thickens.
5. Return the drained pasta to the pot it was cooked in. Remove the bay leaf and toss the sauce with the pasta. Stir over low heat for 1 minute.
6. Salt and pepper to taste and serve immediately.

****Helpful Hint**** At certain times of the year it may be hard to find fresh or canned pumpkin. Substitute butternut squash for the pumpkin. Butternut squash is available all year-round and should be easier to find at your local market.

****Buy and Try**** My new favorite find is Field Roast Sausages, Italian Style. They taste so much like the real thing that people won't believe you when you tell them it doesn't contain any animal products.

14. HEARTY BOWL OF GARBANZO BEANS AND ARTICHOKES

This is one of my favorite protein-packed one-dish meals. It's loaded with fiber, it's grain free, and it's easy to prepare.

Serves 4
Active time: 5 minutes
Start to finish: 20 minutes

Ingredients

> 1 tablespoon olive oil
> 2 (15 oz.) cans garbanzo beans, drained
> 8 sun-dried tomatoes, drained and chopped
> 10 artichoke hearts in water, drained and halved
> 1 teaspoon cumin seeds
> ⅓ cup almond slivers, toasted and ground
> ½ teaspoon salt
> 2 tablespoons lemon juice
> ¼ cup chopped fresh Italian parsley, loosely packed

1. Put the oil in an iron skillet or wok for about 30 seconds on high, until the oil is hot but not smoking. Add in the garbanzo beans and cook for about 10 minutes, stirring just enough so it doesn't burn

but enough that the garbanzos become a nice warm golden brown all over. Place in a large mixing bowl and put aside.

2. Add a smidgen more oil to the pan. Add the sun-dried tomatoes and artichokes and cook until browned. Add the cumin seeds for 1 additional minute. Combine them in a bowl with the garbanzos.

3. Take out a fresh dry skillet and toast the almonds until they turn a light brown color. Put the almonds in a food processor to grind. If you want to save a skillet, place the almonds on a toaster pan for 3–5 minutes. Add the almonds to the artichokes and garbanzos mixture and season them with the salt, lemon juice, and chopped parsley. Serve warm or at room temperature.

****Chef's Secret**** After cooking, wash your wok under hot running water, using a brush to loosen up the food particles. Dry immediately by heating on the stove. Apply a light coat of vegetable oil with a paper towel to prevent your wok from rusting.
****Variation**** Add in white quinoa to really pump up your protein for the day.

15. TERRIFIC TACOS

In my house we have Taco Tuesdays every week. Serve these tasty tacos family style, and everyone gets to create their own taco. Things can get a bit messy, so make sure to have plenty of napkins around for this fiesta!

Serves 4
Active time: 10 minutes
Start to finish: 20 minutes

Ingredients

½ box corn tortilla shells
1 tablespoon olive oil

1 medium onion, diced

2 cloves garlic, minced or pressed

1 package soy crumbles

1 package taco seasoning mix

1 head romaine lettuce leaves (or kale), thinly chopped

2 Roma tomatoes, seeded and diced

½ cup Daiya Cheddar

½ avocado, thinly sliced

½ small red onion, thinly sliced

1 jalapeño chile pepper, finely minced

Fresh cilantro sprigs

¾ cup salsa

6 lime wedges

1. Preheat the oven to 325°F for the tortilla shells.
2. Heat the oil in a medium skillet. Add the onions and sauté for 5–10 minutes, or until the onion becomes soft and translucent. Add the garlic and stir for 1 additional minute.
3. Add the soy crumbles to the onion mix. Continuously stir over low heat until the crumbles have heated up. Be careful as the crumbles can burn easily.
4. Bake the tortilla shells on a baking tray for 5 minutes, or until they become crispy.
5. Put all your fixings on the table and make your own taco!

****Chef's Secret**** When warming up your taco shells, place the open end down on the baking tray. This will stop the shells from closing while heating!

****Buy and Try**** Smart Ground Soy Crumbles. This brand is my favorite, and I love that they now make one with Mexican flavoring.

****Variations**** Substitute the soy crumbles with black beans or pinto beans. This will help keep you full throughout the night.

16. BRAZILIAN BLACK BEAN PATTIES

These hearty bean patties are good standing alone or served like a burger. They are way more delicious then the frozen kind. Kids and adults alike rave about this dish.

Serves 4
Active time: 15 minutes
Start to finish: 45 minutes

Ingredients

⅓ cup tomatillo salsa (or any salsa of your choice)
2 teaspoons ground cumin
½ teaspoon ground coriander
¼ teaspoon minced fresh parsley
¼ teaspoon chili powder
2 (15 oz.) cans black beans, drained
¼ cup green onions, finely chopped
1½ cups whole wheat bread crumbs
½ teaspoon salt
½ teaspoon freshly ground black pepper

For the salsa

2 ripe mangos, peeled and cubed
¼ cup finely chopped red bell pepper
¼ cup finely chopped green bell pepper
1 small green chile pepper, seeded and minced
¼ cup green onions
2 tablespoons chopped fresh cilantro leaves
2 tablespoons fresh lime juice
¼ cup tomatillo salsa
2 teaspoons light agave nectar

1 tablespoon canola oil

½ avocado, cut into ¼-inch dice

1. Preheat the oven to 300°F. In a food processor, mix the salsa, cumin, coriander, parsley, chili powder, and black beans. Blitz the mixture until it is very smooth. Transfer the bean mixture from the food processor and put into a large mixing bowl. With a spatula, fold in the green onions, 1 cup bread crumbs, salt, and pepper. The mix should be evenly combined.
2. Shape the mixture into 8 even patties. In a shallow container, pour in the remaining bread crumbs and dredge each patty. Transfer the patties to a baking sheet and refrigerate for at least 20 minutes.
3. In the meantime, mix together the mangos, peppers, green onions, cilantro, lime juice, salsa, and agave into a small bowl. Chill until serving time.
4. In a large nonstick skillet, heat the canola oil over medium heat. Fry each patty for 3 minutes on each side. Be careful not to let the patties burn. Transfer the patties to a paper towel–lined plate to absorb any excess oil.
5. Keep the patties warm on a baking sheet in the oven and until ready to serve (no longer than 15 minutes).
6. Just before plating, dice the avocado and toss with the mango salsa to combine.
7. Serve 2 patties on each plate, and spoon the mango salsa over the top of each one. Serve immediately.

****Did You Know?**** Many times recipes will call for vegetable oil cooking spray. You probably think to yourself that must be a healthier alternative to using a small amount of oil in your pan. Unfortunately, that may not always be the case. Next time you are at the market, look at the label on the back of a cooking spray can. Notice the serving size and the amount of servings per can. Most cans have upwards of 500 servings, each serving being one third of a second. I don't even really know what one third of a second is. Realistically, how many of you spray your pan for one third of a second? My guess is that you are like everybody else, and you spray your pan in a big circular motion. You have now used 20 to 40 servings of the spray, depending on the size of your pan. So, as you can now see, a small amount of oil in your pan may be the healthier option!

17. COMFORTING CHILI

All chili recipes have changed over time, with new recipes being created every day. If you ask anyone for a chili recipe these days, chances are that you will get a different recipe from every person you ask. My rocking recipe even includes cocoa!

Serves 8
Active time: 20 minutes
Start to finish: 1 hour, 20 minutes

Ingredients

> 1 tablespoon olive oil
> 1 medium onion, diced
> 4 cloves garlic, minced or pressed
> 1 cup sliced mushrooms
> 1 green bell pepper, seeded and cut into ¼-inch dice
> 1 package soy crumbles, crumbled
> 1 cup faux beef stock (I like Better than Bouillon)
> 1 (15 oz.) can red kidney beans, rinsed and drained
> 1 (14 oz.) can diced tomatoes
> 2 cans tomato paste
> 1 tablespoon agave nectar
> 4 tablespoons chili powder
> 2 tablespoons ground cumin
> 2 teaspoons ground oregano
> ½ teaspoon ground coriander
> 2 teaspoons paprika

¼ teaspoon crushed red pepper flakes
½ teaspoon unsweetened cocoa powder
Salt and pepper to taste
½ cup chopped green onions

1. In a large pot or Dutch oven, heat the olive oil over medium heat. Sauté the onion for 5 minutes, or until tender. Stir in the garlic, mushrooms, and bell peppers, and cook for an additional 4 minutes. The onion should now be translucent. Add the soy crumbles and the stock to the onion mixture, and stir to combine for a few more minutes (about 3 minutes).
2. Next to add in are the kidney beans, diced tomatoes, tomato paste, and agave nectar. Continue to stir all the ingredients together until well blended.
3. Add all the seasonings to the pot while continuously stirring. You may need to add some water to the chili at this point, ½ cup at a time. The chili should not be too thick, more of a stew consistency but not as runny as a soup. Remember, some of the liquid will reduce while cooking.
4. Reduce the heat to low, cover, and simmer for at least an hour, stirring occasionally. The longer you let the chili simmer, the more robust the flavors will taste. Check the consistency of your chili after 40 minutes. If the chili is too runny, uncover the pot for the last 20 minutes, or until the desired consistency is reached.
5. Serve into warm bowls and sprinkle the green onions on top to garnish.

****Fun Facts**** Do you know that there are two kinds of tomatoes: one that floats on the water and one that sinks into the water? The tomato that sinks into the water is tastier because it contains more sugar. Do not judge it by color alone.
Also, did you know that if you bring a magnet near the tomato, the magnet will repel? It is because a tomato is 94 percent water, and water molecules repel magnetic fields.

18. FANTASTIC FAJITA SALAD

This is a healthy and fun fajita recipe. By using my culinary instincts and creativity I have made it nutritious and light. You can even make this recipe more tasty and delicious by introducing your own ingredients to it.

Serves 2
Active time: 15 minutes
Start to finish: 45 minutes

Ingredients

1 package Gardein Homestyle Beefless Tips, chopped
¼ cup low-sodium tamari soy sauce
¼ cup fresh lime juice
1 tablespoon olive oil
¼ cup faux chicken stock
1 teaspoon agave nectar
1 teaspoon liquid smoke flavoring
¼ teaspoon hot pepper sauce
2 cloves garlic
2 teaspoons peeled and minced fresh gingerroot
¾ teaspoon ground cumin
½ teaspoon ground oregano
1 large onion, sliced
1 red bell pepper, thinly sliced
1 green bell pepper, thinly sliced
1 head romaine lettuce leaves
½ avocado, diced
Fresh cilantro leaves
Lime wedges
12 cherry tomatoes, halved

1. Defrost the beefless tips for 5–10 minutes.
2. Combine the first 11 ingredients in a jar with a tight-fitting lid and shake well.
3. Cut the tips in half to marinate. Place the beefless tips in a plastic bag or nonmetal baking dish. Pour the marinade mixture over the beefless tips, turning to coat. Seal the bag or cover the dish; marinate at least 30 minutes or 2–3 hours in the refrigerator, turning the tips several times.
4. Remove the beefless tips from the marinade, reserving 2 tablespoons of the marinade. Heat the reserved marinade in a large skillet over medium-high heat. Add the beefless tips, onion, and red and green peppers, searing 3–4 minutes, or until the tips are heated through. Remove from the heat.
5. Line four individual salad plates with the romaine leaves. Spoon the hot mixture over the romaine-lined plates. Top with the avocado and garnish with fresh cilantro leaves, lime wedges, and cherry tomato halves.

****Buy and Try**** Gardein Homestyle Beefless Tips are found at any major food chain in the freezer section. They are a great-tasting product, and super simple to cook with.
****Variations**** If you are feeling like something different, you can easily substitute seitan in this great recipe.

19. CHANNA DAL

Dal is the primary protein source for vegetarians in South Asia and it can also be a great part of any healthy diet. This simple curry is a staple in my house. This recipe is easy, fast, and so tasty!

Serves 4
Active time: 5 minutes
Start to finish: 25 minutes

Ingredients

> 1 tablespoon olive oil
> 1 teaspoon cumin seeds

1 medium onion, finely chopped

2 cloves garlic, minced or pressed

1 tablespoon peeled and minced fresh gingerroot

1 teaspoon seeded and minced green chile pepper

1 teaspoon ground cumin

½ teaspoon turmeric

1 teaspoon ground coriander

2 (14 oz.) cans garbanzo beans, rinsed and drained

1¼ cups faux chicken stock

1 teaspoon garam masala

Salt and pepper to taste

2 tablespoons chopped fresh cilantro leaves

Cooked brown rice (optional)

1. In a medium-size saucepan, heat the oil over medium heat and add the cumin seeds for 1 minute. Add the onion, garlic, ginger, chile pepper, cumin, turmeric, and coriander, and sauté for 2 minutes, stirring constantly.
2. Mix in the garbanzos and the stock and bring to a boil.
3. Reduce the heat to low and cover. Let simmer for 15 minutes. Mix in the garam masala and salt and pepper, and cook for an additional 2 minutes. Remove the saucepan from the heat, and toss the cilantro in with the garbanzo mixture.
4. Serve over brown rice if desired.

****Helpful Hint**** It is always better to use dried beans in a recipe if possible. Cooking dried beans always appears to be a monumental task because it seems like a great deal of time must be spent before you can even use the cooked beans in a recipe. While canned beans are really convenient, cooked dry beans have a lot more flavor than their canned relatives. If you plan ahead, dried beans are easy to cook and are very economical, priced much lower than canned beans. Here is a great tip that will make cooking dried beans easier for you: If you have the freezer space, cook more than one batch of beans at a time. Freeze the cooked beans for up to

6 months. This way you have more flavorful beans but your frozen beans are just as convenient as purchased canned beans.

20. CITRUS GINGER TOFU

The best thing about tofu—besides its nutritional value—is the way it takes on the flavor of your favorite marinade. I love the zesty orange flavor in this recipe. Chinese food doesn't have to be a once-a-week restaurant treat again!

Serves 4
Active time: 30 minutes
Start to finish: 45 minutes

Ingredients

> 1 (16 oz.) package extra-firm tofu, pressed, drained, and
> cut into 8 (¼-inch-thick) slabs
> 2 tablespoons mirin
> 2 tablespoons fresh orange juice
> 2 tablespoons cornstarch
> 1 bunch broccolini, ends trimmed and cut into 4- to
> 5-inch-long thin stalks
> 2 tablespoons low-sodium tamari soy sauce
> 1 teaspoon light agave
> ¼ teaspoon Asian chile paste
> 1 teaspoon orange zest
> ⅓ cup fresh orange juice
> 1 teaspoon toasted sesame oil
> 1 tablespoon canola oil
> 1 teaspoon peeled and minced fresh gingerroot
> 1 clove garlic, minced or pressed

1. Press and drain the tofu.
2. In a small bowl, combine the mirin, 2 tablespoons orange juice, and

cornstarch and blend well. Place the tofu in a single layer in a shallow nonreactive dish. Pour the marinade over the tofu and marinate in the refrigerator for 30 minutes.

3. Put the trimmed broccolini in a large skillet and cover with water. Cover and bring to a boil. Reduce the heat. Simmer the broccolini 5 minutes, until tender and bright green. Drain the broccolini and plunge into an ice bath. Drain and lay the broccolini on a paper towel to dry.

4. In another small bowl, whisk together the tamari, agave, chile paste, orange zest, juice, and toasted sesame oil. Put to the side to use later.

5. Using the skillet from the broccolini, heat the canola oil over medium heat. Add the ginger and garlic and sauté for 1 minute. Add the marinated tofu and stir-fry until golden brown on each side. Add the broccolini for 1 minute more and continue to stir-fry. Mix in the tamari sauce and combine. Cook for an additional 2 minutes, or until the broccolini is heated through.

6. Serve immediately.

****Helpful Hint**** Any major food chain should have an Asian section in their store. It is usually in the condiment aisle, where the dressings and marinades are. Ingredients such as mirin, chile paste, and tamari are pretty standard in most markets. If you can't find them, try to find an Asian market, or buy these staples online.

21. HARVEST ARUGULA SALAD

Every year I look forward to the beautiful fall season and all the glory it offers. I created this recipe after harvesting some of my favorite ingredients, and the result was bliss!

Serves 4
Active time: 25 minutes
Start to finish: 60 minutes

Ingredients

1 teaspoon olive oil

1 small butternut squash, cut in half, seeded and cubed

2 sprigs fresh rosemary, stems removed, plus more for garnish

½ cup red quinoa, rinsed and drained

1 cup water

2 tablespoons raw pumpkin seeds (or pepitas)

2 tablespoons raw sunflower seeds

¼ cup chopped walnuts

4 stalks celery, chopped

1 cucumber, peeled, seeded, and diced

1 Gala apple (or whatever variety you prefer), peeled and diced

4 cups arugula, washed and dried

For the dressing

3 tablespoons balsamic vinegar

1 teaspoon finely minced shallot

1 clove garlic, minced or pressed

1 teaspoon Dijon-style mustard

1 teaspoon agave nectar

½ teaspoon sea salt

¼ teaspoon freshly ground black pepper

¼ cup olive oil

1. Preheat the oven to 425°F. In a small bowl, drizzle the olive oil over the butternut squash and toss to coat evenly. Spread the butternut squash into a single layer over a baking tray. Sprinkle with fresh rosemary, and roast in the oven for 20–25 minutes, or until the squash is tender. Transfer the squash to a plate and chill.

2. Meanwhile, in a small pot, combine the quinoa and water and bring to a boil over medium-high heat. Reduce the heat to low and simmer for 15 minutes, or until all the water is absorbed. Fluff with a fork, transfer to a plate, and chill.

3. While the quinoa is cooking, preheat a toaster oven to 350°F. Line the toaster tray with aluminum foil, and spread the pumpkin seeds, sunflower seeds, and walnuts in a single layer. Cook for 3–5 minutes, or until the seeds and nuts are lightly toasted. Transfer to a plate and let cool.

4. Next make the dressing by blending the balsamic vinegar, shallot, garlic, mustard, agave, salt, and pepper in a blender. With the machine running, gradually add the olive oil through the opening in the lid to process into a thick dressing.

5. In a large salad bowl, toss the celery, cucumber, apple, arugula, chilled squash, chilled quinoa, and a third of the dressing together. You will only need enough dressing to lightly coat the salad. If you feel a third of the dressing isn't enough, add the desired amount. Now add the seeds and walnuts and toss until everything is evenly blended.

6. Divide the salad onto four plates and garnish with rosemary sprigs. Serve promptly.

****Chef's Secret**** When making a green salad, you never want to pour your salad dressing onto your salad until right before you serve it. If you do pour the dressing on and it sits for more than about 15 minutes, you will end up with a salad of mush. On some occasions (picnics, tailgating, potlucks) it may not be appropriate to bring a big salad bowl to toss your dressing into your salad. My secret is to bring the salad in a large ziplock bag and keep the dressing in a separate container. When you are ready to serve, pour your dressing into your ziplock, seal it shut, and shake, shake, shake! You now have a well-tossed salad without the mess.

22. MASOOR DAL

I have been so fortunate to travel the world and sample many different cuisines and cooking methods. This Indian dal is truly an epicurean delight.

Serves 4
Active time: 10 minutes
Start to finish: 40 minutes

Ingredients

> 1 tablespoon cumin seeds
> 1 tablespoon canola oil
> 1 teaspoon poppy seeds
> 1 medium onion, finely diced
> 1 small shallot, minced
> 2 teaspoons very finely minced fresh gingerroot
> 3 cloves garlic, minced or pressed
> 1 red chile, finely diced
> 1 teaspoon turmeric
> 1 teaspoon garam masala
> 2¼ cups red lentils, rinsed and drained
> 1 (14 oz.) can diced tomatoes
> 1 teaspoon agave nectar
> 6 cups vegetable stock
> Cooked brown rice
> ¼ cup roughly chopped raw cashews (optional)
> ¼ cup seedless raisins (optional)
> ¼ cup shredded coconut (optional)
> ¼ cup roughly chopped fresh cilantro leaves (optional)

1. In a large pot, dry roast the cumin seeds for 2–3 minutes over medium heat, or until they become aromatic. Remove from the pan

and grind in a spice grinder. If you don't have a spice grinder, you can mince the seeds with a sharp knife.

2. Using the same pan, turn the heat to high, add the oil and the poppy seeds and cook until the poppy seeds begin to pop. Reduce the heat to medium and sauté the onion and shallot for 2 minutes. Adjust the heat to low and stir in the roasted cumin, ginger, garlic, chile, turmeric, and garam masala, and cook for 1 additional minute, stirring the entire time.

3. Add the red lentils and tomatoes to the spice mixture, and toss to combine. Drizzle the agave over the mixture and increase the heat to medium-high. Add a splash of stock and continue stirring the lentils into the spice mixture for 1 additional minute.

4. Add the remaining stock and bring the dal to a simmer. Reduce the temperature to low and cook, uncovered, for 25 minutes. The dal should be a stew consistency, and the lentils should be nice and soft.

5. I usually serve this over brown rice, which absorbs all the yummy juices from the dal. If you desire, top the dal with the nuts, raisins, coconut, and cilantro leaves, and serve immediately.

****Did You Know?**** Have you ever read a recipe that calls for coriander but then saw the same recipe calling for cilantro? Don't worry; it can be a bit confusing. In the U.S., the seed of the herb is referred to as coriander. So usually coriander is used when a recipe is calling for dried herbs for soups and stews. The stem and leaves are referred to as cilantro. So a recipe calling for cilantro is calling for the fresh green herb used in guacamole and salads.

23. MOROCCAN VEGETABLE TAGINE

Moroccan cuisine is known for its flavorful tagines. A tagine is an exotic stew that has a spicy aroma, and it's very easy to make. This recipe makes a mouthwatering meal every time.

Serves 4
Active time: 15 minutes
Start to finish: 45 minutes

Ingredients

1 tablespoon olive oil
1 small onion, sliced
2 cloves garlic, minced or pressed
½ cup baby carrots
¾ cup eggplant, cut into ½-inch cubes
1 cup zucchini, cut into ½-inch cubes
1 cup red ripe tomatoes, cored and diced
1¼ cups sweet potatoes, cut into ½-inch cubes
¼ cup chopped dried apricots
1 tablespoon fresh lemon juice
1 tablespoon agave nectar
3 cups faux chicken stock (I like No Chicken Base by
    Better Than Bouillon)
¼ teaspoon dried thyme
½ teaspoon ground cinnamon
¼ teaspoon ground cumin
¼ teaspoon ground coriander
1 (15 oz.) can garbanzo beans, rinsed and drained
½ teaspoon salt
¼ teaspoon freshly ground black pepper
Cooked couscous
¼ cup sliced almonds, toasted lightly (optional)

1. In a large heavy pot or Dutch oven, heat the oil over medium-high heat. Sauté the onion and garlic in the oil until tender, about 5 minutes.
2. Mix the carrots, eggplant, zucchini, tomatoes, sweet potatoes, and apricots and combine with the onion mixture. Stir in the lemon

juice, agave, and stock, and season with the thyme, cinnamon, cumin, and coriander. Make sure the stock is covering the vegetables. If necessary, add the appropriate amount of stock. Bring to a boil over high heat, cover, reduce the heat to low, and simmer until the vegetables are tender, about 30 minutes.

3. Add the garbanzos and season with salt and pepper. Stir to combine and cook for an additional 10–15 minutes. Serve over couscous, and sprinkle with almonds if desired.

****Did You Know?**** Research shows that of any food, apricots possess the highest levels and widest variety of carotenoids. Carotenoids are antioxidants that may help to prevent heart disease, reduce "bad" cholesterol levels, and protect against cancer.

24. PENNE PASTA WITH SUN-DRIED TOMATOES

Pasta . . . somehow I never tire of pasta. So many different sauces, so many shapes, so many possibilities. I love the way this pasta is so simple, yet so satisfying.

Serves 2
Active time: 5 minutes
Start to finish: 20 minutes

Ingredients

> 8 ounces rice pasta (I like Tinkyada), cooked according to package directions
> 1 teaspoon olive oil
> 2 cloves garlic
> 1 cup zucchini squash, cut into ¼-inch dice
> ¼ cup sun-dried tomatoes, drained and chopped
> 1 cup broccoli florets
> ¼ cup pesto sauce (recipe on page 237)
> Salt and pepper to taste

2 tablespoons pine nuts (pignoli), toasted

⅓ cup fresh basil leaves, cut into chiffonade

1. Bring a large pot of water to a boil and cook the pasta.
2. Meanwhile, using a large skillet, heat the oil over medium heat. Add the garlic and sauté for 1 minute, or until the garlic becomes fragrant. Garlic burns very easily, so watch it.
3. Add the vegetables to the garlic and sauté for 4 minutes, stirring occasionally. Add the pesto sauce to the vegetable mix and toss until everything is evenly coated with the pesto. Cook for an additional 3 minutes, or until the vegetables are lightly browned and cooked al dente.
4. After the pasta is finished cooking, drain the pasta and return to the pot it was cooked in over low heat. Add the vegetable sauce to the pasta and combine. Season with salt and pepper, and remove from the heat.
5. Divide the pasta evenly between two plates. Sprinkle with pine nuts and place the basil chiffonade in a small mound in the center to garnish. Serve promptly.

****Variations**** I love to put some Kalamata olives and sliced portobello mushrooms in this dish. Then stir in some fresh arugula just before removing from the heat. You can use just about any vegetable you like in this dish. Remember, you want to cook things *you* like to eat, so add your favorite ingredients.

25. PUERTO RICAN SPICY BEAN STEW WITH RICE

Red beans and rice are an important staple in Puerto Rican cuisine. Most of their stews contain bacon for its smoky flavor. In this recipe I add chipotle pepper for that same smokiness, and trust me, your heart will thank you later!

Serves 4
Active time: 20 minutes
Start to finish: 60 minutes

Ingredients

- 1 cup brown basmati rice, rinsed and drained
- 2 cups water
- 1 tablespoon olive oil
- 3 cloves garlic, minced or pressed
- 1 small onion, finely diced
- 2 medium carrots, finely diced
- 1 poblano pepper, finely diced
- 1 green bell pepper, finely diced
- 1 dried chipotle pepper
- ½ cup finely chopped fresh cilantro, plus more for garnish
- 2 (15 oz.) cans red kidney beans, rinsed and drained
- ¼ cup tomato sauce
- ½ teaspoon dried oregano
- ¼ teaspoon ground cumin
- ⅛ teaspoon salt
- ¼ teaspoon freshly ground black pepper
- 2 cups stock (I like Better Than Bouillon No Chicken Base)
- 2 medium Yukon Gold potatoes, cubed
- 1 cup cubed butternut squash

1. Put the brown rice and water in a pot. Season with salt to taste. Set the heat to high and bring to a boil, uncovered. Once it comes to a boil, reduce the heat to low. Cover the pot with a lid wrapped in a kitchen towel to absorb the excess liquid. Simmer on low for 35–45 minutes. Turn off the heat and let the rice sit in the covered pot at least another 10–20 minutes.
2. In the meantime, place the oil in a large saucepan on medium-high heat; heat the oil for 1 minute. Stir in the garlic, onion, carrots, peppers, and cilantro and sauté until the onion is tender, about 5 minutes.
3. Next mix in the beans, tomato sauce, oregano, cumin, salt, and pepper and combine with the onion mixture. Add 2 cups of stock (or

enough stock to cover the beans by 1 inch) and bring to a boil for 4 minutes.

4. Add the cubed potatoes and squash and stir. Reduce the heat to low and simmer, stirring occasionally, for 30 minutes.
5. Divide the rice among four bowls, and place the bean mixture on top. Garnish with cilantro and serve immediately.

****Chef's Secret**** Most people love the nutrition that beans provide, but they are leery of eating them because they get embarrassed from the gas beans cause. Here is a simple way to prevent that: In a stockpot, place 1 pound of beans in 10 or more cups of boiling water. Boil for 2 to 3 minutes. Then cover and set aside overnight. The next day, 75 to 90 percent of the indigestible sugars that cause gas will have dissolved into the soaking water. Drain the soaking water that the beans were in and replace with fresh water to cook in. It is as simple as that.

26. WILD RICE–STUFFED SQUASH

Stuffing squash is a great way to turn this delectable vegetable into a meal. If you can't find an acorn squash for this dish, any winter squash will do.

Serves 4
Active time: 15 minutes
Start to finish: 60 minutes

Ingredients

2 whole acorn squash (or winter squash), cut in half and seeded
1 (15 oz.) can cannellini or navy beans, rinsed and drained
¼ cup faux chicken stock
1 tablespoon olive oil

1 medium onion, finely chopped

2 cloves garlic, minced or pressed

⅓ cup chopped sun-dried tomatoes, drained

2 stalks celery, finely chopped

⅛ teaspoon crushed red pepper flakes

¼ cup faux bacon bits

1 cup wild rice, cooked

2 tablespoons pine nuts (pignoli)

½ cup fresh basil leaves, cut into chiffonade

Salt and pepper to taste

1. Preheat the oven to 400°F. Cut the squash in half and remove the seeds. On a baking pan covered with aluminum foil or a nonstick silicone mat, lay the squash open side down, on the pan. Roast for 20 minutes.

2. In a small bowl, mash ¼ cup of the beans with the stock, and set aside for later.

3. Meanwhile, heat the oil in a large skillet over medium-high heat. Sauté the onion, garlic, sun-dried tomatoes, celery, and red pepper flakes for 5 minutes, or until tender. Toss in the faux bacon bits and cook an additional minute, stirring frequently. Remove from the heat.

4. Stir the mashed beans, whole beans, rice, 1 tablespoon pine nuts, and half of the basil into the skillet, and combine with the vegetable mixture. Season to taste.

5. Using the roasted squash halves, place them on the baking sheet, open side up. Divide the bean and vegetable mixture evenly into the squash, and press the mixture firmly until you have a nice mound on top.

6. Cover the baking pan with aluminum foil and reduce the oven heat to 375°F. Cook the squash for 15 minutes.

7. Uncover the squash and bake for an additional 6 minutes or until the squash and vegetables are lightly golden on top.

8. Use the remaining basil and pine nuts to garnish, and serve promptly.

****Did You Know?**** Acorn squash is a good source of dietary fiber and potassium. Wild rice is an excellent source of protein and is very low in fat. Combine the two, like in the recipe above, and you have a complete meal that will keep you full for hours.

****Buy and Try**** For a great-tasting healthy alternative to bacon bits, try Frontier organic Bac'uns. Use them to top salads, baked potatoes, or your favorite soups. Most supermarkets will carry a vegetarian substitute for bacon bits.

27. THAI GREEN CURRY

I am a huge fan of curries in all forms. In particular, I think Thai curries are bursting with flavor. This green curry paste is just packed with fresh ingredients and it is literally as easy to make as pureeing all the ingredients in a food processor.

Serves 4
Active time: 15 minutes
Start to finish: 60 minutes

Ingredients

- 1 package water-packed extra-firm tofu, pressed, drained, and cubed
- 1 stalk prepared lemongrass [See Helpful Hint]
- 5 cloves garlic
- 1 shallot, chopped
- 2 Thai chiles (jalapeño is a good substitute if you can't find Thai)
- 1 thumb-size piece of fresh gingerroot, peeled and sliced
- ½ cup fresh Thai basil (regular fresh basil works well also)
- ½ cup roughly chopped fresh cilantro sprigs
- ½ teaspoon ground cumin
- ½ teaspoon ground coriander

½ teaspoon ground white pepper

1 teaspoon agave nectar

1 tablespoon fresh lime juice

2 14 oz. cans lite unsweetened coconut milk

1 tablespoon olive oil

1 small yellow onion, cut into ¼-inch dice

1 green pepper, cut into ¼-inch dice

1 red pepper, cut into ¼-inch dice

1 small zucchini, diced

1 cup sweet potato, cut into ½-inch cubes

1 cup broccoli florets

1 cup fresh snow pea pods

½ 14 oz. can bamboo shoots (or an entire 8 oz. can), drained

Cooked brown basmati rice, ⅓ cup per serving

1. Press the tofu and drain for at least 20 minutes to release all the excess water.
2. In the meantime, make your green curry paste. In a food processor or blender, mix the prepared lemongrass, garlic, shallot, chiles, ginger, basil, cilantro, cumin, coriander, white pepper, agave, lime juice, and ¼ can of the coconut milk. Set aside the remaining coconut milk to use later. Blitz well to make a fragrant green curry paste.
3. In a large pot, add the olive oil and heat over medium heat for 1 minute. Sauté the onion for 5 minutes, stirring occasionally. Add the cubed tofu and vegetables, and continue to sauté for an additional 2–3 minutes. You want the vegetables to remain firm. Pour the remaining coconut milk into the pot. Next stir in the curry paste slowly to get a nice smooth sauce. Reduce the heat to low and simmer for at least 20 minutes.
4. Serve the curry in warm bowls atop brown basmati rice.

****Helpful Hint**** You can find fresh lemongrass in most Asian food and grocery stores. Look in your local grocery store in the specialty produce department. When buying fresh lemongrass, look for stalks that are fragrant and tightly formed.

To prepare fresh lemongrass, you want to use the softer, fleshier part of the lemongrass. This is located under the tough outer leaves. Peel away the outer layers with your fingers and discard. Using a sharp knife, cut off the lower bulb about 2 inches from the bottom of the stalk and discard. Now it should be fairly easy to cut up the lemongrass. Starting from the lower end (where the bulb was) make thin slices up to two thirds of the stalk. Now place the sliced lemongrass in a food processor and pulse five times. You have just prepared your lemongrass.

****Variations**** This is a great dish to prepare when you are cleaning out your refrigerator. Use all the fresh veggies you have left over from your week. This curry tastes great with just about any vegetable you can imagine, and you can even use frozen vegetables to make this easy dish. This is a great lunch to take to work the next day, so don't throw out any leftovers!

28. TROPICAL BEAN STEW

This black bean stew recipe is very appetizing and very filling. I love the fruitiness of the mango against the rich black beans and the mild blend of spices.

Serves 4
Active time: 10 minutes
Start to finish: 35 minutes

Ingredients

    1 tablespoon olive oil
    1 medium onion, chopped
    ½ cup green onions, chopped
    2 cloves garlic, minced or pressed
    1 green pepper, cut into ½-inch dice
    1 red pepper, cut into ½-inch dice
    1 jalapeño pepper, seeded and minced

2 medium sweet potatoes, cut into ½-inch dice

1 (14 oz.) can diced tomatoes, drained

¾ cup vegetable stock

2 (15 oz.) cans black beans, rinsed and drained

1 ripe plantain (or banana), sliced ½ inch thick

1 ripe mango, peeled and diced

½ cup chopped fresh cilantro leaves

2 tablespoons shredded coconut for garnish

1. Heat the oil in a large pot or saucepan over medium heat for about 1 minute. Add the onion and green onions and sauté for 5–7 minutes, or until tender. Add the garlic for an additional minute and stir until fragrant.
2. Mix the peppers, sweet potatoes, tomatoes, and stock into the pot, and bring to a boil.
3. Reduce the heat to low and simmer for about 20 minutes. You want the sweet potatoes to still be firm.
4. Add the beans and continue to simmer, uncovered. Cook for 5 minutes. The beans should be heated through.
5. Stir in the plantain, mango, and half of the cilantro, and gently stir until everything is heated through.
6. Sprinkle the coconut and remaining cilantro over the beans to garnish.

****Helpful Hint**** To pick a plantain that is ripe, look for one that is yellow and black in color. The more black it has on the skin, the sweeter it will taste. A healthy way to prepare a plantain is to steam it. With the skin on, cut off the top and the bottom ends of the plantain, and make a long slit down the entire length of the fruit. Next cut the plantain into 3 equal pieces, and put in a steamer basket over hot water. Steam for 10 to 15 minutes, or until the fruit is bright yellow and soft. A well-ripened plantain will cook faster, so time accordingly. ****Did You Know**** What is the difference between a banana and a plantain, you might ask. Plantains tend to be firmer and lower in sugar content then bananas. Both fruits are a great source of potassium and dietary fiber, but they are consumed a bit differently. Bananas are almost always eaten raw, while plantains tend to be steamed, boiled, grilled, baked, or fried.

29. CHICK'N WITH CREAMY MUSHROOM SAUCE

The Gardein Chick'n Scallopini is a staple I always have in my freezer. Use it just like you would use a chicken breast and create lots of different meals. You can change the sauce, grill them, chop them, and put them on a salad. You're the chef!

Serves 4
Active time: 15 minutes
Start to finish: 35 minutes

Ingredients

> 1 cup gluten-free flour (I like Bob's Red Mill)
> 1 package Gardein frozen Chick'n Scaloppini (do not thaw)
> 1 tablespoon olive oil

For the mushroom sauce

> 1 tablespoon olive oil
> 1 small onion, finely chopped
> ¾ cup sliced white mushrooms, stems removed
> ¾ cup sliced wild mushrooms (use any kind you want or just double the white mushrooms), stems removed
> 3 cloves garlic, minced or pressed
> ½ cup white wine
> ⅓ cup faux chicken stock
> ⅓ cup cashew cream (page 120)
> 1 teaspoon Earth Balance buttery spread

½ teaspoon dried thyme (or fresh if you have it)
Salt and pepper to taste

1. Pour the flour into a shallow container. Lightly dredge the chick'n in the flour. In a large nonstick skillet, heat the oil over medium-high heat. Sauté each chick'n patty for 2–3 minutes on each side, or until lightly browned. Transfer to a baking tray and put in a 200°F oven while you make the sauce.
2. In the skillet you used to cook the chick'n, heat the oil over medium heat. Add the chopped onion and sauté for 5 minutes, or until tender. Add the mushrooms and cook for 3 more minutes. Next add the garlic and sauté until fragrant, about 1 minute.
3. Pour in the white wine and bring the mixture to a boil. Reduce the sauce by about half. Pour in the stock and gently whisk in the cashew cream. Bring the sauce to a boil again, and cook for 4–5 minutes, or until the sauce has thickened.
4. Stir in the Earth Balance and let melt. Stir in the thyme and salt and pepper, taste, and stir to combine.
5. Place the chick'n onto four plates and pour the mushroom sauce over; serve immediately.

****Chef's Secret**** Steer clear of table salt, which is more processed and contains added ingredients. Use kosher salt or sea salt instead.

30. CAPRESE PANINI

Italian cuisine is a very important aspect of Italian culture. The Caprese salad is a highly famed staple of Italian cuisine, greatly loved and imitated all over the world. I decided to step it up a notch and turn it into a heavenly sandwich.

Serves 2
Active time: 15 minutes
Start to finish: 15 minutes

Ingredients

> 4 tablespoons pesto sauce (page 237)
> 4 slices Ezekiel 4:9 bread (or other multigrain bread)
> 4 thin slices tomato
> Salt and freshly ground pepper to taste
> 4 fresh basil leaves
> ½ cup loosely packed arugula leaves
> 4 slices mozzarella cheese substitute (I like Daiya brand)
> 2 teaspoons olive oil
> 2 teaspoons balsamic vinegar

1. Spread 2 tablespoons of pesto on top of a slice of bread. Next, lay tomato slices on the pesto. Sprinkle the tomatoes with salt and pepper. Place the basil and arugula leaves on top. Finally the mozzarella should be the last layer on the sandwich. On another slice of bread, drizzle one side with olive oil and balsamic vinegar, and place the bread, oil side down, to create the sandwich.
2. Cook the sandwich in the panini press set on medium-high heat. The sandwich is ready when the cheese is melted, about 6 minutes. If you don't have a panini press, cook the sandwich on a grill pan or in your toaster oven.
3. Repeat for the other sandwich.

****Did You Know?**** The proper way to store olive oil is in a dark, room-temperature cupboard or even in the refrigerator. The healthy nutrients in olive oil as well as the taste can slowly degrade over time, so it's probably best to use it within a year or within six months once opened.

SIDE DISHES

1. MASHED SWEET POTATOES

Yummmm . . . Everyone loves mashed potatoes. Let's face it: they are the ultimate comfort food. Traditional mashed potato recipes are made with loads of butter, cream, and salt. These mashed potatoes are just as yummy and good for you!

Serves 4
Active time: 5 minutes
Start to finish: 40 minutes

Ingredients

> 6 medium sweet potatoes, peeled and diced (5 cups)
> 1 tablespoon Earth Balance
> ⅓ cup cashew cream (page 120)
> 1 tablespoon agave nectar
> ¼ teaspoon ground cinnamon
> Salt and freshly ground pepper to taste

1. Place the potatoes in a large pot and cover them with water. Bring to a boil over high heat and cook, uncovered. Once the water is boiling, cook for 10–12 minutes, or until tender. Drain the potatoes.
2. Transfer the potatoes to a large mixing bowl. Using the whisk attachment, mix the potatoes for 1 minute on low speed. Add the Earth Balance, cashew cream, agave, and cinnamon. Whip on medium-high until very smooth. Season with salt and pepper, and whip 1 additional minute.
3. Serve immediately.

****Did You Know?**** Besides being simple starches, sweet potatoes are rich in complex carbohydrates, dietary fiber, beta-carotene, vitamin C, and vitamin B_6.

2. ORANGE BROCCOLI

This broccoli dish will give you a double dose of your daily vitamin C.

Serves 2
Active time: 5 minutes
Start to finish: 15 minutes

Ingredients

> 1 teaspoon olive oil
> ¼ bag frozen broccoli
> 2 cloves garlic, minced or pressed
> ⅓ cup orange juice
> 1 tablespoon orange zest

1. Place the oil in a large nonstick skillet over medium-high heat.
2. Add the broccoli and stir-fry for 3 minutes or until lightly browned.
3. Add the garlic to the pan and cook for 1 additional minute.
4. Decrease the heat to medium-low, pour the orange juice over the broccoli, and cover the pan.
5. Let the juice steam the broccoli until the broccoli is tender, about 5 minutes.
6. Sprinkle the zest over the broccoli and serve immediately.

****Chef's Secret**** Looking for a way to reduce your oil while cooking? I learned several years ago that you only need a small amount of oil to cook most foods. I have a technique you might want to try and see if it works for you. First you want to make sure the pan you are about to use is not hot. I put 1 tablespoon of oil in my pan. I swish that oil around the best I can. Next, I wrap a paper towel or paper napkin around two fingers, my pointer and middle finger. I put my wrapped fingers in the oil and rub the pan in a circular motion until the pan is evenly coated with the oil from my paper towel. You will notice the paper towel has absorbed quite a bit of the oil in the pan. Now your pan is evenly coated with a much smaller amount of oil then you started with!

3. ROASTED ASPARAGUS

Recipes don't have to be complicated to be tasty. This is a perfect example of the less-is-more theory.

Serves 2
Active time: 5 minutes
Start to finish: 15 minutes

Ingredients

> ½ pound asparagus, tough ends snapped off
> 1 tablespoon olive oil
> Sea salt
> Freshly ground pepper

1. Preheat the oven to 400°F.
2. Place the asparagus in a single layer in a roasting pan.
3. Drizzle the asparagus with the oil and toss to evenly coat the spears. You can also hand roll the asparagus along the extra oil on the bottom of your pan.
4. Sprinkle with sea salt and pepper.
5. Roast until the spears are tender and lightly browned, 10–15 minutes.

****Variation**** After the asparagus is cooked, drizzle 1 tablespoon of balsamic vinegar over the spears for a nice tangy flavor.

4. SWEET ROASTED CARROTS

I was never a fan of cooked carrots until I created this recipe. They always brought back memories of the carrots I had at the cafeteria in grade school. They were mushy and flavorless. Now I know that roasting carrots brings out their natural sweetness and they are actually yummy! Who knew?

Serves 2
Active time: 5 minutes
Start to finish: 40 minutes

Ingredients

> 8 whole carrots
> 1 tablespoon olive oil
> 1 tablespoon chopped fresh rosemary leaves
> Salt and pepper to taste

1. Preheat the oven to 400°F.
2. Trim the tops and bottoms off the carrots and peel. Cut in half lengthwise.
3. In a small roasting pan, place the carrots in a single layer. Drizzle with olive oil and roll the carrots back and forth on the pan. This will help evenly coat both sides of the carrot.
4. Sprinkle with the rosemary and salt and pepper, again rolling the carrots back and forth on the pan to get seasonings on both sides.
5. Bake for 30–40 minutes (the roasting time will vary depending on the thickness of your carrot), turning the carrots over halfway through.
6. Carrots are best when they are browned on all sides and soft.

****Buy and Try**** I honestly do not know how people can live without a Silpat nonstick baking mat. Silpat is a silicone mat designed to fit your baking pans and cookie sheets. The mat allows you to never have to grease a pan again! I use my Silpat every time I put anything in the oven. The amazing thing about a Silpat is that nothing sticks to it so it makes your cleanup so much faster. Plus you can reduce the amount of oil you use in your recipes and you can help save the planet by never having to use parchment paper again. They're available in any cooking store or on Amazon.com.
****Variation**** You can use just about any fresh herb when roasting carrots. My favorites are thyme and sage. This carrot dish is a great accompaniment to any holiday meal.

5. SESAME ASIAN SLAW

Traditionally, coleslaw has been a mayonnaise-based salad. This coleslaw is bursting with flavor, easy to make, and is anything but traditional.

Serves 4
Active time: 10 minutes
Start to finish: 25 minutes

Ingredients

¼ cup rice vinegar
1 teaspoon olive oil
1 teaspoon toasted sesame oil
1 tablespoon low-sodium tamari soy sauce
1 tablespoon agave nectar
1 clove garlic, minced or pressed
¼ teaspoon red pepper flakes
3 green onions, sliced
½ cup seeded and diced cucumber
1 cup grated red cabbage
1 cup grated green cabbage
2 medium carrots, grated
1 tablespoon chopped fresh cilantro
2 tablespoons chopped fresh basil
1 tablespoon toasted sesame seeds

1. In a small mixing bowl, combine the rice vinegar, oils, tamari, agave, garlic, and red pepper flakes. Cover the bowl and refrigerate 20 minutes.
2. In a large mixing bowl, combine the onions, cucumber, cabbages, carrots, cilantro, and basil.
3. Combine the salad and dressing, and toss just before serving.
4. Sprinkle sesame seeds on top to garnish.

****Time-saving Tip**** Most supermarkets sell the grated cabbage and carrot mix in a 16-ounce bag. Less mess, less time, and same great taste.

6. CREAM OF BROCCOLI SOUP

This homemade recipe is much better than anything from a can. This sophisticated broccoli soup is rich and creamy, plus it has the added goodness of spinach. People don't think of serving soup as a main course, but there's no reason not to—not when it's creamy good like this!

Serves 4
Active time: 30 minutes
Start to finish: 1½ hours

Ingredients

1 tablespoon olive oil
1 medium onion, chopped
1 leek, sliced, white and pale green section only
2 stalks celery, chopped
1½ pounds broccoli, florets chopped, stems trimmed
    and chopped
2 cloves garlic, minced or pressed
2 quarts faux chicken stock
1 bay leaf
½ teaspoon salt
¼ teaspoon freshly ground pepper
1 cup cashew cream (page 120)
2 cups fresh spinach
2 roasted red peppers (optional)

1. Heat the oil in a heavy stockpot over medium-high heat. Add the onion, leek, and celery and sauté for 6 minutes, or until the onion

is tender. Add the broccoli and sauté for 8 minutes. Add the garlic and continue to sauté the mixture for an additional minute, or until fragrant. Stir in the stock, bay leaf, salt, and pepper, and bring to a boil. Now reduce the heat to low and simmer for 25 minutes. Add the cashew cream and simmer for an additional 10 minutes. Discard the bay leaf.

2. Working in batches, pour the soup into the blender about three quarters of the way full. Puree. Add the spinach to the very last batch and continue to blend until the spinach is a smooth puree. Pour all the soup, other than the spinach batch, back into the pot. Finally stir in the spinach batch to combine. Serve in soup bowls.

3. If desired, in a food processor puree the roasted peppers with 1 tablespoon cashew cream, and blend until smooth and creamy. Drizzle on top of the soup for garnish.

****Variations**** You can use just about any green vegetable to make this delicious soup. I love it with asparagus.

DESSERTS

1. CHOCOLATE-COVERED STRAWBERRIES

This is the world's most decadent and simplest dessert that you will ever make. Whenever I serve them at a dinner party, people are so impressed! If they only knew that they take only 10 minutes to make. Shhh . . . our little secret!

Serves 4
Active time: 10 minutes
Start to finish: 10 minutes

Ingredients

12 long-stemmed whole strawberries
½ cup vegan dark baking chocolate

1. Prepare a baking sheet by lining it with parchment paper or a Silpat baking mat.
2. Wash the strawberries and dry them thoroughly.
3. In the top of a double boiler over boiling water, melt the chocolate, stirring occasionally, until the chocolate is smooth. Turn off heat.
4. Holding a strawberry by the stem, dip it in chocolate, rolling in a circular motion to evenly coat most of the berry. Let the excess chocolate drip from the strawberry back into the pan.
5. Carefully transfer each strawberry to a baking sheet.
6. Chill in the refrigerator for 15 minutes to set the chocolate before serving.

****Buy and Try*** Find a dark chocolate with a high cocoa content. Endangered Species makes a great bar called All Natural Extreme Dark. It has 88 percent cocoa content in it. Scharffen Berger also has bittersweet chocolate baking chunks with 70 percent cocoa. Try and stay away from the vegan chocolate chips if possible, as they contain a lot of sugar.

****Variation**** If you want to spice things up a bit, you can top your strawberries with a variety of ingredients. After dipping your berry, roll it in crushed almonds or pistachios. If you are really feeling adventurous, add ⅛ teaspoon ground chili powder to the melted chocolate before you dip your berry. The options are endless . . .

2. CHOCOLATE MOUSSE WITH RASPBERRY COULIS

This chocolate mousse recipe is simple to make and virtually foolproof. The mousse has a rich chocolate flavor and is light and velvety smooth, almost like pudding. It will even satisfy the hard-core chocolate lovers!

Serves 4
Active time: 10 minutes
Start to finish: 40 minutes

Ingredients

> 12 ounces silken soft tofu (I like Mori-Nu tofu, in the
> small cardboard box)
> 2 ounces vegan dark baking chocolate (I like the
> Endangered Species All Natural Extreme Dark
> chocolate bar)
> 1 teaspoon vanilla extract
> 2 tablespoons agave nectar
> 1 pint fresh or frozen raspberries
> 1 tablespoon lemon juice

1. Melt the chocolate over a double boiler, stirring constantly.
2. In a food processor or Vitamix, combine the tofu, chocolate, vanilla and 1 tablespoon of agave nectar and blend. Make sure to occasionally scrape the sides of the bowl. Blend for 2 minutes.
3. Transfer the mousse to individual cups. (I love to use martini glasses for this.)
4. Chill in the refrigerator for 30 minutes.
5. In the meantime, purée the raspberries, remaining agave nectar, and lemon juice in a blender until smooth.
6. Using the back of a large spoon, press the puree through a fine-mesh sieve into a bowl to remove the seeds.
7. Pour the raspberry mix over the mousse just before serving.

*****Variation**** You can flavor this mousse several different ways by just adding 1 teaspoon of mint, coconut, or orange extract to the tofu mixture before blending. The raspberry coulis is optional; I use it as a "wow" factor when serving guests.

3. SILKY STRAWBERRY PUDDING

This blissful dessert is ridiculously easy to make, with some seriously impressive results. Wow your guests when you bring this out—they will think you have been in the kitchen for hours!

Serves 4
Active time: 5 minutes
Start to finish: 1 hour, 5 minutes

Ingredients

> 8 ounces frozen strawberries, unsweetened, thawed and
>   drained
> 12 ounces firm or extra-firm silken tofu (I like Mori-Nu)
> 1 tablespoon orange zest
> ¼ cup agave nectar (optional)
> 1 tablespoon vanilla extract
> 4 fresh strawberries, sliced

1. In a food processor, combine all the ingredients except the sliced strawberries, stopping after 1 minute to scrape the sides of the bowl.
2. Blend for an additional minute or until the mix is very smooth.
3. Divide the mix evenly among small bowls, and chill for at least 1 hour.
4. Garnish with sliced strawberries and serve immediately.

****Variations**** Substitute the strawberries with your favorite fruit, and make this recipe your own. My personal favorites are raspberry with orange zest or mango with lime zest.
****Buy and Try**** Mori-Nu silken tofu is probably the most recognized brand of tofu. Check your grocer's dry foods section to find it (it comes in a small cardboard box and does not require refrigeration). Ask your grocer if he carries Mori-Nu silken Lite Tofu, or ask him to order it for you. The Lite Tofu is just as yummy as the regular tofu, just fewer calories!

4. SIMPLY SWEET FRESH FRUIT

There are some days when I just need to satisfy my sweet tooth but I don't want to make a big fuss. This recipe does the trick.

Serves 4
Active time: 10 minutes
Start to finish: 10 minutes

Ingredients

   4 tablespoons cashew cream (page 120)
   1 pint fresh strawberries, sliced
   1 tablespoon orange zest
   1 tablespoon agave nectar

1. On a small dessert plate, dollop 1 tablespoon cashew cream in the middle of the plate. Don't spread the cream too thin, just enough to make it the size of a silver dollar.
2. Using a quarter of the strawberries, place the slices on top of the cashew cream.
3. Sprinkle a little bit of the orange zest over the strawberries.
4. Drizzle a quarter of the agave nectar on top.

****Variation**** Omit the orange zest from the recipe and replace it with shredded coconut.

Shopping and Resource Basics

Here are some basic things to help you shop and eat well. Remember to just lean in to all this, and don't make yourself crazy. Take a weekend afternoon and wander a health food store, a farmers' market, and the healthier part of your local grocery (the periphery aisles where the produce is and the "health foods" aisle if they have one).

   Once you're in the swing of things, I'd suggest you always go grocery shopping with a complete list of what you need and don't get anything other than what you've itemized. And don't go shopping when you are hungry (impulse buys can be deadly)!

Proteins

Try to have a protein at every meal; this way your diet is sure to be balanced, and you'll feel energetic and strong.

Tofu is bean curd, soy. It has very little flavor so it can be used in either savory or sweet dishes and will take on the flavor of whatever sauce or seasoning you use. It's low in calories, cholesterol, and fat, and it's high in protein and iron. You'll find it near cheese or in the "fresh" section of markets.

If you think you don't like tofu, listen to what my reader Yvonne had to say:

TOFU. Just the word brings up images of crazy, crunchy hippies. I bought the container and let it sit in my fridge until it expired. Then I did it again. I knew I wanted to try it, but I really didn't know how. Finally I read a description that changed my mind. It said something along the lines of, "You can't not like tofu. It's like saying you don't like flour. No one eats a handful of flour and no one eats a plain slice of tofu. It's an ingredient, and you find the recipes you like. If you don't like the outcome, you try it in something else, as you would most other ingredients." Okay, so I had to find a recipe. I found one for vegan lasagna, and the tofu was blended with olive oil, garlic, and salt. It was supposed to mimic the ricotta cheese. I liked that it could be "hidden" in a lot of yummy Italian layers. Pasta and garlic, how could I go wrong? I still used my tofu ricotta sparingly in the layers, just in case. Well, I loved it! And so did my husband. He didn't even know he was eating a vegan meal! I had put ground imitation meat [texturized vegetable protein, or TVP, which you can find in your grocery store] in the sauce along with onions and mushrooms. Well, now I was really onto something. I could trick people! So I had my dear old dad over for leftovers, and he loved it! Success!

Tempeh is made from cultured soybeans, which are formed into a sort of cake. It's easily digestible, has a nutty flavor, and is very high in protein, dietary fiber, and vitamins. It has a stronger flavor than tofu. It's usually found near the cheese section.

Seitan is made from wheat gluten and is chewy in texture. It is high in protein, very low in fat, and is extremely versatile in cooking. Nearly anything made with meat can be made with seitan instead. Find it near the cheese or vegan section of your market.

Beans and legumes are high in complex carbohydrates (the good kind!), fiber, iron, and folic acid; they also have a lot of protein. You can store them in your pantry almost indefinitely, and use them for bean salads, soups, and casseroles: black beans, lentils, garbanzo beans, lima beans, adzuki beans, black-eyed peas, edamame, fava beans. Beans are my protein of choice; they are super healthy, so opt for them often! Canned are also fine; just rinse them first to get rid of the salt!

Nuts and seeds and nut butters have plenty of fiber, nutrients, and antioxidants along with healthy monounsaturated fats; nuts and seeds go far in filling you up and making you feel satiated. Try almonds, cashews, walnuts, pecans, pistachios; almond butter, peanut butter, tahini, and so on. Choose raw and unsweetened, with no salt. My new favorite brand is PB2 powdered peanut butter; it's got all the protein of peanut butter but without all the oil. It's kind of perfect!

High-protein meat alternatives are wonderful transitional proteins as you move away from meat and toward plant-based options. They are delicious, but I recommend eating whole foods as often as you can. Things that grow in the ground or on trees are what you want to fill your diet with. Still, I believe in progress, not perfection!

Gardein Garden+Protein: These high-protein, center-of-the-plate meat alternatives are delicious and easy to prepare as an entrée or an ingredient in a soup, stew, sandwich, or whatever. Gardein is my absolute favorite alternative meat, as it tastes so good and my meat-eating friends always love it. I recommend the Beefless Tips, which are great for stew or on a skewer with other veggies, and Chick 'n Scallopini, which you can use in any way you would use chicken; it's highly versatile and easy to cook with. *www.gardein.com*

Tofurky: I love their Italian Deli Slices for sandwiches. They also make several flavors and styles of tempeh. Their holiday "turkey" looks like sliced turkey, so you can enjoy the feast along with everyone else at the table. *www.tofurky.com*

Field Roast: These folks make two of my favorite products. Celebration Loaf is a vegan "roast" with mushroom stuffing; it's a nice presentation for holiday or special events and great with a homemade sauce or gravy. Also their Field Roast Sausages are the best and come in several different flavors. I like the Italian and serve it with portobello mushrooms, red peppers, fennel root, tomatoes, and garlic over pasta. *www.fieldroast.com*

Nate's Meatless Meatballs: Add them to a pasta sauce, or sauté, stick a toothpick in it, and *voilà*, a delicious appetizer. Now you can add "meatballs" to anything!

Lightlife Smart Ground meatless meat crumbles are great to use in tacos, chili, or any sort of meat sauce. I serve them to hearty eaters as well as kids all the time, and they never know they aren't eating meat! *www.lightlife.com*

Starches

Whole grains: brown or wild rice, millet, quinoa, amaranth, buckwheat, corn, et cetera.
Sweet potatoes, yams, roasting potatoes
Flax crackers, rice cakes
Steel-cut oats and whole grain hot cereal mixes

Whole grain breads (try the sprouted ones, and go for gluten-free if you are sensitive to gluten). Most whole wheat is still pretty processed, so try rye and pumpernickel. My favorite is Manna bread, which you can find in health food stores, if not some mainstream grocery stores.

Whole grain pastas made from artichoke, corn, quinoa, spelt, black beans, or brown rice. (This last is my favorite; it looks and tastes like regular white pasta. Be sure not to cook it too long, and you may want to rinse it with cold water before you put the sauce on.)

Vegetables and Fruits

Squashes, broccoli, kale, mustard greens, Swiss chard, spinach, cucumbers, carrots, radishes, dried figs, apples, plums, blood oranges, tomatoes, artichokes, cauliflower, brussels sprouts, eggplant, all kinds of mushrooms, salad greens, cherries, blueberries, limes. You get the drift; whatever looks fresh and colorful, give it a whirl. Steer clear of sweetened dried fruits.

Vegetarian Cooking Stocks and Broths

> Imagine Foods No Chicken Broth
> Imagine Foods Vegetable Stock
> Pacific Organic Mushroom Broth
> Pacific Organic Vegetable Broth
> Rapunzel Bouillon Cubes
> Better Than Bouillon No Beef
> Better Than Bouillon No Chicken Base

Nondairy

Cheeses: These are several companies whose products I use and enjoy. My favorite is Daiya because it tastes and melts just like cheese. See *www.daiyafoods.com*.

Again, these cheeses are part of "leaning in." They should be used sparingly and as a treat while you move ever more toward whole foods that grow in the ground or on trees. They have fat and calories to consider, so please use them as transitional foods to make your lean comfortable.

Soya Kaas, Sunergia Soy Foods (*www.sunergiasoyfoods.com*), Follow Your Heart (*www.imEarthKind.com*), and Galaxy Nutritional Foods (*www.galaxyfoods.com*) are all good, and come in Cheddar, mozzarella, Parmesan, and feta. Follow Your Heart is what I use for eggplant Parmesan and hot paninis.

I like Silk Soy Creamer to mix into hot beverages. It's rich and delicious. Use only a tad, as it has sugar and fat. It's better than milk or cream, though, which is why I'm compromising a bit here.

Instead of cow's milk, try hemp, rice, almond, or soy milk. Get them unsweetened, and use stevia to sweeten to taste.

Cream cheese and sour cream: Tofutti (*www.tofutti.com*). Tofutti cream cheese has 4 grams less fat in a 2-tablespoon serving size compared with regular cream cheese, plus 4 grams less saturated fat and absolutely no cholesterol. Follow Your Heart Cream Cheese has 2 grams of fiber and no trans fats, even though it has more calories and fat, so it too is a good alternative.

Butter: Earth Balance Natural Buttery Spread. This is a tasty substitute for butter, but use sparingly, only when no other substitute works.

Pantry / Staples

Follow Your Heart Reduced Fat Vegenaise mayonnaise substitute. It has lower total fat than regular mayo; it's very low in saturated fat, has no cholesterol, and has no hydrogenated or partially hydrogenated fat and no trans fats. Use it sparingly!

Condiments: Ketchup, mustard, relish. Annie's Naturals are some of the best I've found. (*www.anniesnaturals.com*). Also, Cascadian Farm and Woodstock Farms are good (*www.cascadianfarm.com*).

Canned goods: Pasta sauces, beans, and vegetables. Try Eden Organic (*www.edenfoods.com*), Muir Glen (*www.muirglen.com*), and Walnut Acres Organic (*www.walnutacres.com*). Good products. I love the Muir Glen Fire Roasted Diced Tomatoes!

Oils: Use extra-virgin olive oil and canola—and sparingly. You can use the sprays, too, but remember: a very small spray!

Egg substitute: Ener-G Egg Replacer. It's nothing more than potato starch and tapioca starch mixed into a powder, to which you add water, and it works really beautifully for baking (*www.ener-g.com*).

Keeping the Cost Down

I know getting healthy food is sometimes challenging and expensive, but it doesn't have to be. You just have to know where to look! Leaning in to a healthy diet can actually help you save on food bills.

1. Buy in season. Produce in season is almost always less expensive than out-of-season produce because it's more abundant.

2. Avoid precut, washed, and packaged fruits and vegetables. They're always more expensive than the whole foods (and a waste of packaging). If you need the convenience, go for it; just know that you'll be paying more.

3. Watch produce prices carefully. Locally grown fruits and vegetables sometimes cost less than imported produce, while at other times imported produce saves you a lot—just be on the lookout for the best deals. (And be mindful of the carbon footprint—how far your food had to travel to you and therefore how much fuel was required to get it there.)

4. Shop at farmers' markets at the end of the day. Farmers' markets are a great place to find fresh, in-season, and locally grown produce for cheap—especially if you shop at the end of the market day when growers may be willing to sell their produce at a discount, rather than have to pack it up and take it back home with them.

5. Don't be afraid to buy frozen vegetables. Frozen veggies (especially store brands) are often cheaper than fresh ones, and they can actually be *more* nutritious because the veggies are frozen right after they're picked, preserving vitamins that are lost in transporting fresh veggies from the farm to the store. And of course, keep an eye out for sales and stock up your freezer with

veggies that can be tossed into soups, stews, stir-fries, pasta, and many other dishes.

> **Extra Lean:** If you are making a soup or casserole, make twice what you need and freeze the rest so that you have some ready-made meals for the weeks to come.

6. Consider the value of your time. For most of us, time is just as valuable as money. We tend to think that eating fast food is less time consuming—an illusion reinforced by a steady stream of fast-food company advertising. But in reality, the time you spend driving to a fast-food restaurant and then idling in a drive-through could just as easily be spent at home with your family, cooking a simple meal. All it takes is a small initial time investment in learning to cook a few new meals. Even simpler, you can just convert the meals you already eat into ones that fit your new lifestyle.

Most families rotate the same menu of dishes every week, for ease of preparation and to simplify grocery shopping. Once you've got that set menu of favorite meals, prep time is quick.

Definitely check out the big bulk stores like Sam's Club or Costco. They have big frozen bags of veggies you can stock up on and load into your freezer. You could even split bulk buys of beans/rice/grains/veggies with friends.

Some health food stores will sell the 50-pound bags of grains and dried beans if you ask, and may give you a good price if you order them in advance.

A great online site, *BulkWholeFoods.com*, has many great dried bulk foods, grains, and rice.

Amazon sells beans and grains as well—just search on *www.amazon.com*.

Here's a very handy little guide to the cheapest fruits and veggies by the month, to help you save money: http://frugalliving .about.com/od/foodsavings/tp/Cheapest_Produce.htm

And here are some more resources you might find useful. (Thanks, Natala, for your list!)

Some Great Resources to Check Out

Recipe Sites
    http://blog.fatfreevegan.com
    http://simplifiedfood.com
    http://happyherbivore.com
    http://veganyumyum.com
    http://vegandad.blogspot.com
    http://kblog.lunchboxbunch.com
    http://therealmealtoday.blogspot.com
    http://www.managercomplete.com/engine2/recipes.aspx
    http://fatfreevegan.com
    http://www.holycowvegan.net
    http://chocolatecoveredkatie.com
    http://vegweb.com

Guided Meditations
I have some on my website, www.kathyfreston.com/ and they are also offered on Amazon and iTunes.

Great Recipe Books
    The 30-Minute Vegan by Mark Reinfield and Jennifer Murray
    1,000 Vegan Recipes by Robin Robertson
    Appetite for Reduction by Isa Chandra Moskowitz
    Color Me Vegan by Colleen Patrick Goudreau
    The Complete Guide to Vegan Food Substitutions by Celine Steen and Joni Marie Newman
    Eat, Drink & Be Vegan by Dreena Burton
    Eat Vegan on $4 a Day by Ellen Jaffe Jones
    Forks over Knives: The Plant-Based Way to Health by Gene Stone
    The Get Healthy, Go Vegan Cookbook by Dr. Neal Barnard

The Gluten-Free Vegan by Susan O'Brien
The Happy Herbivore Cookbook by Lindsay Nixon
More Great Good Dairy-Free Desserts Naturally by Fran
    Costigan
Party Vegan by Robin Robertson
Unprocessed by Abbie Jay
Vegan Family Meals: Real Food for Everyone by Ann Gentry
Vegan Lunch Box by Jennifer McCann
Vegan on the Cheap by Robin Robertson
The Vegan Slow Cooker by Kathy Hester
Vegan Soul Kitchen by Bryant Terry
The Vegan Table by Colleen Patrick Goudreau
Veganomicon by Isa Chandra Moskowitz and Terry Hope
    Romero
Viva Vegan! by Terry Hope Romero

Healthy Eating Out
http://happycow.net
http://www.vegdining.com/Home.cfm
http://www.vegetarianusa.com
http://www.vegguide.org
http://www.vrg.org/travel

There are also vegan/vegetarian groups in almost every major city, so you can go online to find out what's near you. It's great support as you continue to lean in.

Phone Apps (to help you find good food wherever you go)
Cruelty Free
Everyday Vegan
ilocate Vegan Restaurants
iVegetarian
PCRM 21 Day Vegan Kickstart
Vegan Is Easy
Vegan Recipes

Vegan YumYum
VeganSteven
VeganXPress
Vegetarian Smartlist
Veggie Passport
Veggie Spots
VegOut
VegWeb /Vegan Recipe Finder

Great Health Books

Veganist: Lose Weight, Get Healthy, Change the World by
   yours truly; I had to include these!
The Quantum Wellness Cleanse by yours truly yet again
Breaking the Food Seduction by Neal D. Barnard, M.D.
*The Cancer Survivor's Guide: Foods That Help You Fight
   Back* by Neal D. Barnard, M.D.
The China Study by T. Colin Campbell, Ph.D.
* Dr. T. Colin Campbell has an excellent certification program
   through Cornell University on plant-based nutrition.
Cholesterol Protection for Life by Joel Fuhrman, M.D.
Disease-Proof Your Child by Joel Fuhrman, M.D.
Dr. McDougall's Digestive Tune-Up by John A.
   McDougall, M.D.
Eat for Health by Joel Fuhrman, M.D.
Eat to Live by Joel Fuhrman, M.D.
The End of Overeating by David A. Kessler, M.D.
The Food Revolution by John Robbins
Foods That Fight Pain by Neal D. Barnard, M.D.
The Get Healthy, Go Vegan Cookbook by Neal D. Barnard, M.D.,
   and Robyn Webb
Mad Cowboy by Howard F. Lyman
The McDougall Program by John A. McDougall, M.D.
The McDougall Program for Maximum Weight Loss by
   John A. McDougall, M.D.
The Pleasure Trap by Douglas J. Lisle, Ph.D.

Prevent and Reverse Heart Disease by Caldwell B.
Esselstyn, Jr., M.D.

Films and DVDs to Watch for Day 21, Connect the Dots

45 Days: The Life & Death of a Broiler Chicken, by Compassion Over Killing. This will show you what happens in the brief life of chickens, who are slaughtered at just 45 days old. You can find it at *ChickenIndustry.com.*

Earthlings, narrated by Joaquin Phoenix. This one is widely hailed as the best documentary about the treatment of animals in society, and it's also the one video on this list that covers more than the meat industry.

Farm to Fridge, narrated by James Cromwell (yes, from *Babe*!). Cromwell explains precisely what happens to animals—from the farm to the fridge—and it has already been viewed more than a million times. See it at *MeatVideo.com.*

Free Range: A Short Documentary. To better understand labels like "free range" or "humanely raised," watch this video to see what happens on the "best of the best" meat ranches.

Glass Walls, narrated by Sir Paul McCartney. In this film, McCartney gives slaughterhouses (and factory farms) glass walls: he narrates, animal by animal, precisely what happens in modern food production. **If you're going to watch just one video, I suggest this one.** You can find it online at *Meat.org.*

Meet Your Meat, narrated by Alec Baldwin. This is probably the most famous behind-the-scenes video ever, and has been viewed millions of times at *MeetYourMeat.com.*

Mercy for Animals Investigations. This is not one video; it's 13 shorts (and it will surely be more by the time you read this), which will give you a good, clear look at what happens to animals as they become food. Find it at *MercyforAnimals.org/investigations.*

Overlooked: The Lives of Animals Raised for Food by the Humane Society of the United States. This is an eye-opening look at the modern meat industry. Go to *HSUS.org*, or search online for the title.

Health and Cooking Videos
Chef AJ and Dr. Matt—Healthy Made Delicious
Fat, Sick, and Nearly Dead
Forks over Knives
Processed People
Sugar: The Bitter Truth
Tackling Diabetes with Dr. Neal Barnard

Health-Related Websites
http://engine2.org
http://www.heartattackproof.com
http://pcrm.org
http://www.rawfor30days.com/index4.html
http://www.tcolincampbell.org
http://www.NutritionFacts.org

Recipe Index

General Index

ACE (American Council on Exercise), 150
aerobic (cardiovascular) exercise, 79, 145, 148–49, 151, 153
agave, 34, 50, 166, 169, 170, 171, 172
ALA (alpha-linolenic acid), 72
alcohol, 51–52
almonds, 27, 127
American College of Sports Medicine, 151
American Dietetic Association, 66, 129
amino acids, 123, 128–29
Anderson, James W., 58–59
animal products, 35–36, 57–67, 122–34, 221–22
  antibiotics in, 73
  body weight and, 89, 131–32
  cholesterol in, 12–13
  cravings and, 64–65
  dairy, *see* dairy products
  dinner and, 122–34
  eggs, 12–13, 63, 73, 128, 156, 158, 167, 220, 221
  fat in, 14, 61, 64–65, 92–93
  fiber and, 10, 14, 63
  fish, 57, 63, 65, 158
  lunch and, 57–67
  meat, *see* meat
  poultry, *see* poultry
  production of, and ethics, 156–60
  viruses in, 10
anthocyanins, 75, 103
antibiotics, 73, 75
antioxidants, 53, 99, 100, 101, 103, 104, 114
  catechin, 55–56
anxiety, 79, 84
appetite, 114, 163
  chocolate and, 100
  coffee and, 53
  fiber and, 41
  nuts and, 27, 28, 31
  protein and, 123
apples, 15–20, 171
  anti-cancer properties of, 16
  fiber in, 16–17, 19–20
arginine, 29–30
Atkins diet, 58–59, 189, 221

weight training, *see* strength
training
Whelan, Elizabeth, 60
Willett, Walter, 126, 220
willpower, 156, 157

yams, 191, 226
yeast, nutritional, 105

zinc, 100
Zone diet, 59–60

Acknowledgments

I HAVE SO ENJOYED WRITING THIS BOOK, BUT IT HAS IN NO WAY BEEN A solo adventure. I have been truly lucky and blessed to have such brilliant and skillful people helping me pull this work together.

To begin with, big gratitude goes to the team at Weinstein and Perseus Books: Harvey Weinstein, John Radziewicz, Katie McHugh, and Amanda Murray. And a special thanks to David Steinberger who has personally championed my books since we began our partnership. I am a creature of comfort, and this publishing family has become such a comfortable and friendly home for me.

Thanks to Jennifer Rudolph Walsh, my agent at William Morris Endeavor, who has always helped hone and streamline my ideas. She knows my heart and my intentions, and keeps nudging me forward. I rest easy knowing she has my back.

Thanks to Emily Votruba for her careful copyediting. Ellen Rosenblatt for making the typesetting easy on the eye.

I so appreciate Brian Chojnowski and Alex Camlin for the cover design, which really speaks to the ease of this Lean plan.

A big hug to Heidi Bassett Blair, my dear friend who swung into action and photographed me one day after hiking, when I realized we needed a fresh new photo for the book cover.

Huge thanks to Stacy Davies and Nicki Graham for their research and contributions.

To Neal Barnard, MD and Michael Greger, MD who shared with me their expertise and peer reviewed data I needed to make sure the Lean plan is medically sound—I am in awe of their knowledge.

And a hearty thank you goes to chef Dayna McLeod for the delicious recipes included in the book; her dishes make leaning in super simple and delicious.

And once again, warmest gratitude to my adored editor Caroline Pincus; I could not have written this book without her. She is the shapeshifter of manuscripts, a shaman of words.

Finally, a deep bow to the many people who shared their stories of weight loss in the pages herein; they did the work and are living testimonials of how a shift in diet can profoundly change your life for the better. I am forever in awe of those who rise to their challenges and triumph.